THE SOCIAL CONTEXT OF DENTISTRY

The Social Context of Dentistry

Peter Davis

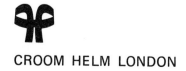

CROOM HELM LONDON

© 1980 Peter Davis
Croom Helm Ltd. 2-10 St John's Road, London SW11

British Library Cataloguing in Publication Data

Davis, Peter
    The social context of dentistry.
    1. Dentistry – Social aspects
    I. Title
    301.5   RK51.5

ISBN 0-7099-0512-6

Printed and bound in Great Britain by
Biddles Ltd, Guildford and King's Lynn

CONTENTS

ACKNOWLEDGEMENTS

The library research for this book, together with the first draft, were completed while I was on sabbatical leave from the University of Auckland. My thanks to the university for its support during this period. While in London I benefited from discussions with a number of people, especially Aubrey Sheiham (of the London Hospital Medical College Dental School) and Giles Dussault (of Bedford College, Social Research Unit). I also had access to the unrivalled collection of material at the British Dental Association Library. Thanks are also due to Rosamund Sarfas for her editorial work on the manuscript, and to the various people on 'the fifth floor' who allowed me to use their typewriters at different times.

ACRONYMS

The following acronyms have been used in the text:

ADA	American Dental Association
AMA	American Medical Association
BDA	British Dental Association
DHSS	Department of Health and Social Security
DMF	Decayed, Missing and Filled
GNP	Gross National Product
HBM	Health Beliefs Model
IADR	International Association of Dental Research
UK	United Kingdom
USA	United States of America
USPHS	United States Public Health Service
USSR	Union of Soviet Socialist Republics
WHO	World Health Organisation

For Helen

1 DENTISTRY IN SOCIETY

From Artisan to Professional

In a little over a hundred and fifty years dentistry has developed from the ill-organised endeavours of a band of itinerant tooth-drawers operating on the fringes of a precarious personal service economy, to an established, respected and powerful occupational group that has taken a central place in the burgeoning health sector of the advanced industrial societies. At the beginning of this period dentistry was still practised very much as a secondary occupation. The great majority of dentists were tradesmen who advertised their wares and worked in an itinerant manner, or from a shop, combining their dental work with other service activities such as selling medicaments, wig-making, hair-cutting and minor surgery (Richards, 1968: 137-41). Indeed, it is clear from commentaries of the time, that the dentist was regarded as somebody exercising a rather limited range of skills. 'An artisan, who confines himself to the extraction of teeth and to several operations required by their defects' was one definition current at the time. And, as if the artisan status of the occupation were still in doubt in the reader's mind, the commentary goes on to add that 'the head surgeons in London deem this branch of their art beneath notice and generally decline interfering in it'.[1] Moreover, this image of the dentist-as-artisan persisted well into the nineteenth century; as late as 1849 a dentist is still defined rather restrictively as 'one who cleans and extracts teeth', according to an entry in a current dictionary,[2] an image that lingers on in the popular mythology of modern dentistry.

Yet, in a little over a century since these words were written, the transformation of dentistry has been complete. What was once a poorly-organised, itinerant trade has since become a powerful and prestigious profession. Indeed, on a number of measures of the organisational strength of the profession such as size of membership, wealth and expertise, and on various criteria of internal unity such as the homogeneity, stability and involvement of its membership, dentistry clearly rivals medicine in the forefront of the modern health professions; in some respects the dental profession is probably more united and better integrated than any other occupation in the health field, at least in the United States (USA) (Akers and Quinney, 1968).

Perhaps more striking than the change over the last century or so is the transformation of the occupation that has taken place over little more than a generation since the 1920s. From an occupation riven by internal divisions, held in low public esteem and providing little more than the traditional artisan services of extraction, reconstruction and minor repair, dentistry has, in the course of thirty years, become an independent, united and respected profession that, in its technical accomplishments and in its philosophy of client care, stands in many ways as the prototype health occupation in the modern personal service sector. As recently as the 1920s, dentistry was still regarded by most commentators as a mechanical art rather than a health profession. Gies, whose report to the Carnegie Foundation in 1926 was to usher in the major reforms of dental education in the USA, argued that dentistry was still predominantly the art of realigning, repairing, rebuilding and removing teeth, a mechanical art of restoration rather than a branch of medicine. It was this tradition that Gies sought to bring to an end by eliminating apprenticeship training in dentistry and by introducing the basic medical sciences into the dental curriculum (Gies, 1926:3-18).

This same tradition of mechanical dentistry in North America had been roundly denounced by William Hunter, the British surgeon, a decade before. Like Gies, Hunter attacked the undue emphasis placed on elaborate reconstructive work, work that was often carried out with scant regard for the oral condition and usually in ignorance of the broader principles of medical science (Gullett, 1971: 124). Conditions were little different in the United Kingdom where, as in other trades, the majority of dentists learnt their skills by apprenticeship. As late as 1918, the 'unqualified' or apprenticed practitioners outnumbered by two-to-one those dentists who had received some formal education (Carr-Saunders and Wilson, 1933: 111), a situation that lagged behind the USA where practitioners with formal qualifications were in a majority by the turn of the century (Gies, 1926: 45). Yet, barely a generation later, with the legal and educational restrictions on entry into the profession which followed in the wake of various reports and which responded to pressure from the dental practitioners themselves, dentistry had clearly emerged in the public consciousness as a skilled, white-collar occupation with a status close to that of medicine. While the 1920s were clearly a transition period, with an occupation of uncertain public standing and very mixed social recruitment and composition, by the 1950s dentistry was drawing new recruits largely from the elite and enjoyed an unchallenged standing as an occupation of professional status.[3]

Certainly, the rapidity and apparent discontinuity of such a change in the fortunes and public image of an occupation should not be overdrawn. After all, in many respects the impression of continuity is just as striking as the signs of change. Not only is the occupation still largely a male preserve (at least, outside the Nordic and East European countries where the proportion of women in the profession can be anything up to 90 per cent (Allred, 1977: 30)), but the predominant unit of service remains the solo practitioner. Furthermore, then as now, a major though declining proportion of dental services still consists of the extraction of teeth and the fitting of dentures. Moreover, we know that, by the end of the eighteenth century, figures such as Fauchard in France with his classic text, *Le Chirurgien Dentiste,* and Hunter in England *(A Practical Treatise on the Diseases of the Teeth)* had made significant advances in attempting to place the dental experience of their day on a more systematic and scientific basis (Menzies Campbell, 1958).

Therefore, there is in dentistry a distinct scientific and medical tradition that provides a further strand of continuity between its occupational origins and its emergence as a profession. However, while there may be elements of continuity in the organisation and even the content of dental work, and while it is quite possible to detect signs of a self-conscious professional identity in the early days of dentistry, the transformation of medieval barber-surgeon, first to skilled tradesman, and then to modern professional, remains a striking testament to the rapidity with which social institutions can change and provides an impressive example of the opportunities for social movement afforded by the industrial revolution and the emergence of the market economy.

The Growth of the Service Sector

This short chronicle of one occupation's progress from trade to profession is not in any way unique to dentistry, though the rapidity of the transformation is remarkable by any standards. In fact, far from being unique, the rise of dentistry can be seen as part of a much broader movement involving the expansion of the entire service sector in industrial society. This development has been quite a general one in the advanced industrial economies and has been characterised by a number of changes in the area of the production and distribution of services. In the first place, a growing share of resources has been allocated to this sector (including the social and personal services), with a corresponding decline in the importance of the manufacturing sector. Secondly, there has been continuous development of a complex occupational structure, with the institutionalisation of scientific and technical advancement in universities and research institutes and the widespread application of such expertise in industry and the social services.

Although it has been argued by some commentators that these features of the so-called 'service economy' are more particularly, perhaps uniquely, characteristic of the highly industrialised societies and reflect a 'post-industrial' stage of growth,[4] there is considerable evidence that the service sector has witnessed rapid and almost unchecked economic growth since the earliest stages of industrialisation. It is evident, for example, that the proportion of the work-force employed both in agriculture and the service sector has always been greater than the manufacturing portion of industry for as long as reliable statistics are available (Kumar, 1976: 445).

Therefore, while the personal service economy in which dentists participated in the early-nineteenth century may have been fluid and precarious, and while dentistry may largely have been a secondary occupation that was rarely practised on its own, the provision of personal dental services was one area of occupational specialisation among many in what was a much broader and rapidly expanding service sector that had its pre-industrial origins in the flourishing craft guilds of the Middle Ages. The demand for services continued to grow apace through the early stages of industrialisation; rather than it being the case that manufacturing expanded at the cost of the service sector — in fact it was agriculture that declined — it was, on the contrary, the growth of industry that provided the all-important boost to the market for personal services. Economic advancement and changes in occupational structure led to a growing urban middle class and a stable and more prosperous working-class who could reasonably aspire to the services of the modern practitioner.[5]

In the twentieth century the service sector has expanded particularly rapidly. Castells (1976: 596) estimates that, in the case of the USA, the number of workers employed in the production of goods has been virtually static over the period 1940-68, while the service sector has, by contrast, doubled in size. Indeed, the USA is the first and, at present, only society in which the number of white-collar workers exceeds the number employed in manual work,[6] a fact that provides a measure of the growing importance of the service sector and that, given the social class-related nature of the market for professional services, also gives a rough indication of the potential level of demand in this area.

According to Castells, growth has occurred in the commercial services such as trade, finance, insurance and real estate, and also in government employment, but not in the personal services. What growth there has been in the social services has taken place in the 'semi-professional' area — white-collar workers, less highly qualified than those in elite occupations, and largely employed in the public service sector in health, education and welfare (Kumar, 1976: 451-2). Recent figures for the USA, for example, show that employment in these areas has increased 69 per cent over the period 1960-70, compared to a growth of less than 20 per cent in employment in the manufacturing sector (Stevenson, 1978: 455). Yet, the personal service sector *has* expanded, as has the employment of more highly qualified white-collar workers. Halmos (1969: 32-3), for example, argues that there has been a significant expansion of professional employment. On his calculations the proportion of professionals in the work-force has increased about threefold in the UK since the turn of the century. Within this group, however, it has to be noted that personal service professionals have multiplied less rapidly than those employed in engineering and in scientific and technical services.

Whilst the growth of the service sector has proceeded virtually unchecked since the earliest stages of industrialisation, the personal service professions like law, medicine and dentistry probably experienced a once-and-for-all increase in size at some early stage before legislative restrictions on entry into the market were introduced. After this period any expansion that took place was more likely to be in allied 'semi-professions' and other ancillaries. Medicine, at least, seems to conform to this pattern. By the turn of the century the great expansion in the medical profession had taken place and by this time had been successfully halted with the introduction of various legal restrictions on entry into the profession. This first stage was rather delayed in the case of dentistry since, in both the UK and the USA, the number of dental practitioners continued to grow unchecked well after the turn of the century. While there were 1,200 qualified practitioners in the UK in 1879 and more than three times that number unqualified, by 1918 there were 4,000 fully qualified dentists and double that number operating without formal qualifications (Carr-Saunders and Wilson, 1933: 111).

In the USA the number of dentists grew by 40 per cent over the decade 1910-20, while the increase in population size was only 15 per cent. By contrast, the number of medical practitioners remained virtually unchanged, largely because of the introduction of formal educational requirements aided by the closure of the proprietary medical schools (Gies, 1926: 83). By the 1940s in all advanced industrial societies progress towards the unification of the dental profession was complete, and the exclusion, or regularisation, of unqualified practitioners had been secured. In this respect therefore dentistry followed quite closely the pattern established in the development of the medical profession, albeit at a distance of, say, two generations.

A crucial agency in helping to secure the closure of the market and the introduction of formal, legislative restrictions on entry into the profession was the state. It was only by state intervention that potential competitors could be eliminated or controlled, the uncertain status of the unqualified regularised and a viable occupational monopoly established. The state played an all-important part in achieving these goals; having played its part, however, the state was then expected to yield its interventionist role and retire from the scene, leaving the professions free to organise their market at will. But this was not to be. Certainly, the state in most cases largely withdrew from any active intervention in the delivery of professional services once occupational monoplies had been established. In time, however, the state was drawn into a more active role, which it has never since relinquished, and has become vitally involved in the evolution of the market for health services.

The nineteenth century was the heyday of *laissez-faire* social philosophies and it was in this period that the market for certain personal services such as dentistry and medicine reached a size and stability in the advanced economies sufficient to support an independent profession charging freely for its services. The role of the state in achieving this market independence was minimal and was largely restricted to the passing of the necessary enabling legislation.

The twentieth century, however, has witnessed a dramatic change in the role of the state and, with it, a greater public interest in the affairs of the health sector. A number of factors have been at play here. Most important, perhaps, has been the emergence in the political arena of a distinct working-class constituency that has sought to advance its principal social goals through the agency of direct state intervention. This has resulted in a growing state commitment in the personal service sector which, together with rising public expectations and developments within the professions, has lead to a dramatic growth in the allocation of resources. In the UK, for example, public expenditure on health, education and welfare more than doubled over the period 1961-73, a rate of increase four times the growth in industrial output in the same period (Draper *et al.*, 1976: 15).[7] Around the same time the proportion of US federal spending allocated to health, education and welfare doubled from 18 to 36 per cent (Iglehart, 1978: 57). In all cases the growth of the health sector has been particularly rapid, with the percentage of the Gross National Product (GNP) allotted to health expenditure doubling in most countries from about three to six per cent over the period 1950-70 (Maxwell, 1974: 18).

The Expansion of Health Services

This development in the health sector is a significant one. In the first place, in Western market economies the growth of the health sector has been associated with the increasing involvement of a number of agencies, e.g. insurance companies, business corporations, unions and, above all, the state. From the time of the first social security health scheme, initiated by Bismarck in Germany in 1883 (Fereday, 1970: 89), the principle of state involvement in the financing of health care had been accepted in most European countries by the outbreak of the First World War, and in many South American states by the 1940s (Roemer, 1971: 354). Even in the USA, where *laissez-faire* and free market principles have reigned largely unchallenged, the American Medical Association (AMA) was on the point of endorsing a compulsory health insurance scheme in 1916; by 1922, however, the mood had changed and since that date the profession has been largely instrumental in blocking any further legislative initiatives in this direction (Numbers, 1978: 110). In the period 1916-18 sixteen states introduced compulsory health insurance bills, but none were enacted and in 1935 major concessions made on the Social Security Act restricted its impact to the area of income-transfer, thus bypassing the health field almost entirely (Anderson, 1971: 110). Nevertheless, the involvement of the state *has* increased in the USA, with the share of health expenditure from public sources growing from 22 to 36 per cent over the five years 1966-71; dental care, however, remains overwhelmingly privately funded (Young, 1974: 45-6).

In the fully developed social insurance systems of Western Europe the proportion of GNP absorbed by social security payments hovers around 15 per cent, with dental care taking anything up to 10 per cent of the sum allocated to health (Groot, 1972: 481). The British National Health Service (NHS) is financed from tax revenues, and not social security contributions; out of the total health budget, dental care absorbs approximately 5 per cent (Lennon, 1978: 481). An alternative route to third-party payment has been followed in the USA where there has been a notable growth in private dental insurance programmes since the Second World War. The number of people covered by dental insurance has increased rapidly from one million in 1962 to over 13 million in 1974, about 15 per cent of the population (Schoen, 1978: 179).

The ifrst important feature of the rapid growth in the health sector, especially since the Second World War, has been the development of indirect or third-party mechanisms to finance personal health services. The simple market model of an atomised and fragmented clientele organised and serviced at will by a single occupational group is therefore a thing of the past, though in many societies dentistry is still much closer than medicine to this earlier form of market organisation. The primary agency for change here has been the state. In part, the growing role of the state in the financing of the health sector has resulted from the pressures of various political constituencies, especially the mass parties of the Left,[8] but a crucial aspect of the increasing involvement of the state has been its wider responsibilities in the economy, particularly in the management of demand and the control of inflation.

The second important point about the growth of the health sector is that, whatever we might infer from the success of the health professions in promoting their occupational concerns, the prominence of health issues in advanced industrial societies tells us much about rising aspirations and expectations of life. Once basic material requirements have been met, as they have for the great majority in the advanced economies, issues of personal health increasingly become debatable points where the great public questions that centre on the security and well-being of the individual are discussed. This is the theme that has been taken up by Renee Fox (1977: 14-15) in arguing that the modern health sector now has a much broader cultural significance that takes it beyond any narrowly-technical definition of the medical task. She claims that while health cannot be said to have any broader cosmic significance of the sort it had in pre-modern society, it does at least touch upon a wider range of moral and social concerns. Hence, on Fox's argument, the rising percentage of GNP allocated to health is only in part attributable to the persuasion of the professions or to the pressures of corporate groups interested in expanding the market for health commodities; in part it must also be attributed to the broadening social signficance of health concerns and the role that health has come to play as a widely-accepted measure of individual well-being.

The idea that the growth of the health sector might have a wider cultural significance, reflecting broader social aspirations rather than the narrower interests of professions or corporate groups, is a proposition

that it is almost impossible to test in any conclusive way. The evidence
on this can only be circumstantial, relating in the main to the expansion
of the medical domain to incorporate ever broader areas of life such as
mental health, sexuality, abortion, birth, death, the management of
stress and so on. Historically, these were areas that once concerned
other agencies such as organised religion, the law, and informal social
mechanisms within the community and the immediate family. Such
matters are now increasingly the subject of medical concern, though
how much this can be attributed to professional self-advancement and
how much to broader humanitarian concerns and changing social standards it is impossible to say.

The notion that these developments can at least in part be associated
with wider cultural changes receives some support from the (admittedly
limited) evidence that people may now place higher expectations on
their personal health than they would have done even a decade ago. For
example, over the 15-year period 1954-69, the number of certificated
days absent from work due to sickness rose 38 per cent in the UK, an
increase which could only in part be attributed to the changing size and
age composition of the insured population concerned (Whitehead, 1971:
20-1). In reporting these figures Whitehead argues that the increase is not
due to any uncovering of further 'objective' health needs, but instead
must be accounted for by changing attitudes to health, especially attitudes to working when sick. Data from other European countries
suggest that these developments are part of a broader trend and that the
increase in sick days in the UK is by no means unusual, and is exceeded
in several of the other countries surveyed (Taylor, 1969: 705).

Health Needs and Patterns of Practice

This question of the relationship between professional interests and
broader social needs and aspirations has a much wider significance than
this discussion of the expansion of the health sector might suggest. In
fact, it goes right to the heart of the relationship between the health
professions and the community at large and raises crucial issues about
the future direction of health services. Nowhere is this more clearly seen
than in the disjunction between health needs and dominant patterns of
professional practice. While the pattern of illness and death in the
advanced industrial societies has quite clearly shifted from acute disorders of the infectious and communicable diseases to chronic conditions that are affected in the main by social factors, the trend within

medicine has been towards high-technology, hospital-based interventions
of a type associated with the tasks of life-saving and curative medicine
rather than with the more mundane tasks of prevention, care and health
maintenance.

In part this shift in the pattern of ill-health, and the associated change
in the social need for health care, is due to the ageing demographic structure of the advanced industrial societies; in Europe, for example, for the
majority of countries the proportion of the population over the age of
60 varies between 15 and 20 per cent (WHO (Copenhagen), 1973: 188).
But a much more important factor, though obviously one related to the
ageing demographic structure, has been the decline in the importance of
the infectious diseases and a corresponding increase in the chronic disorders, not just for the elderly, but over the entire age range. It is these
disorders that have been termed the 'diseases of civilisation', health
problems associated with aspects of industrial society, especially nutritional patterns, the environment, urbanisation, and the pace of social
and economic change. Burkitt (1973) has identified twelve of the most
important of these diseases of affluence, including dental caries, and has
linked their growing prominence in the pattern of illness and death to
specific changes in the modern diet at the turn of the century, as well as
to broader aspects of modern economic development.

Although there is limited evidence for the pattern of morbidity
associated with the 'diseases of civilisation', because information of this
sort is rarely collected in a systematic fashion for total populations, the
statistics on mortality are compelling. Taking deaths due to heart disease,
strokes and cancer alone, in 1969 in the economically advanced countries
of Europe these accounted for 60-70 per cent of total mortality (WHO
(Copenhagen), 1973: 189). Adding just two more causes of death —
chronic bronchitis and diabetes — brings this proportion up to 70-80 per
cent. In other words, for the advanced industrial societies of the world,
just five disorders account for about three-quarters of the total mortality burden. Yet, despite this predominance of chronic, degenerative disorders, the more dramatic and more glamorous aspects of the medical
task continue to dominate the popular imagination, as they tend also to
govern the medical curriculum, medical thinking generally and the entire
reward structure of the profession itself.

Dentistry, by contrast, has always been associated with the treatment
of chronic disorders; one of them, caries (tooth decay), dependent on
diet, and the other, periodontal or gum disease, a condition related
mainly to oral hygiene. Although caries is more clearly a disorder of
modern diet and life style, and hence a classic degenerative disease of the

advanced industrial societies, it is in fact periodontal disease that has upset the traditional mode of practice in dentistry, in much the same way that the growing prominence of the chronic disorders has overturned the orthodox pattern of curative medicine. As a growing proportion of the population keep their natural teeth into adulthood, so the effects of periodontal disease as a potential source of tooth loss become more apparent. Furthermore, because, like caries, it can be controlled but, unlike caries, it cannot be repaired, periodontal disease requires something more than the reparative and treatment philosophy that has been the hallmark of the orthodox approach to dental care (O'Shea, 1971b: 23).

Recent evidence from the World Health Organisation (WHO) suggests that nearly all adults have either gingivitis, a milder gum disease or periodontitis (a more severe form), and often both, and that these conditions are the major source of tooth loss for those over the age of 30 (WHO, 1978: 9). Yet, while the predominant pattern of oral disorder among adults is shifting from the teeth (the dentition) to the gums (the supporting soft tissue), the great majority of professional activities are still those of mechanical and reconstructive dentistry, rather than the tasks of cleaning and prevention (prophylaxis), oral hygiene instruction and routine health maintenance. Although wide use is made of auxiliaries in dental practice, these are in the main deployed to aid the dentist with conventional conservative procedures and tend not to be used in the type of preventive work where they have been shown to be very successful. In a recent review of the use of auxiliaries in Europe it was reported that 30 per cent of the countries surveyed permitted only the employment of laboratory technicians and dental chairside assistants. Although a number of the countries did have preventive workers such as hygienists, the number of such workers actually employed was very small (Allred, 1977:20). Survey data from the recent WHO International Collaborative Study (WHO/ICS) also show a predominantly restorative style of dental practice, with no more than 6 to 7 per cent of practice time spent on oral diagnosis and health education, and much the same again on periodontics (Bonito and Cohen, 1978). Again, it is the mechanical and reconstructive aspects of the dentist's task that persist in the public image of the profession.[9]

Nevertheless, in its organisation of work and in its philosophy of care, dentistry is far more closely attuned than medicine to the requirements of health promotion and health maintenance imposed by the chronic, degenerative disorders that now constitute the bulk of the health burden in the advanced industrial societies. The point about the chronic diseases is that the traditional, curative skills of medical practice are of little avail since, by the very nature of such disorders, their impact is cumulative and largely irreversible. Therefore, to follow a curative philosophy in such instances is to permit a chronic condition to run its course and to develop to a stage where medical intervention may no longer be of any value. The fact, for example, that heart disease is the major killer of men in the 35-64 age group merely reflects the prevalence of a chronic condition which, if left to run its course, may result in disability and premature death. In other words, like the oral condition, which is susceptible both to normal ageing effects and also to the onslaughts of oral disease, the heart and other organs of the body are subject to the degenerative effects of the ageing process and to the impact of the physical and social environment. But, while the dominant technology and philosophy of the heart specialist have been those of acute medicine and various curative procedures, dentistry is more clearly geared, in philosophy if not also in practice, to the concepts of prevention, regular health maintenance and incremental care.

In fact, dental caries may reasonably lay claim to being the first acknowledged 'disease of civilisation' since its association with affluence and 'good living' has long been recognised and is largely beyond dispute (Sognnaes, 1949: 16). The increased consumption of sugar that mainly accounts for the high caries incidence of the advanced industrial societies is well-documented; on recent estimates the world production of sugar has increased fivefold this century, over a period in which the world's population only doubled in size. The increase in sugar consumption has been particularly rapid since the 1940s, as has the growing tendency for the consumption of sucrose to be in the form of manufactured and processed foods, rather than as a household additive (Newbrun and Frostell, 1978: 69). In the advanced industrial societies these trends were well under way before the turn of the century. By the late-nineteenth century there is evidence of a high-caries prevalence in the UK, the USA, Scandinavia and Australasia, and in a number of these countries state authorities instituted special dental services in the schools in order to meet the problem of gross, untreated decay (Burt, 1978: 273).

To this day the Nordic countries tend to have more lavish programmes of dental care, in part because they are in a better position to afford the heavy cost, but also because of this history of high-caries prevalence (Kostlan, 1974: 71). Yet the costs of a full treatment programme are enormous. Suffice it to say that the requirements of care for a single part of the body — the mouth — absorb anything between 5 and 10 per cent of total health expenditure in the advanced industrial societies (Stamm, 1978: 415) and that anything between a third and a sixth of university-trained medical manpower are dentists (WHO (Copenhagen), 1972: 124). In the Nordic countries the ratio lies somewhere between two and three medical practitioners per dentist, and in most remaining industrial societies – apart from the socialist countries – the ratio is between three and five to one. Although the extent of specialisation in dentistry does not match that achieved in medicine, nor is ever likely to – in the USA, where specialisation has gone the furthest, 90 per cent of active dentists are still general practitioners (McCallum, 1978: 399) – the number of auxiliaries per dentist is not very different from the ratio of nursing staff to medical practitioners. Medicine, however, commands a much greater share of resources and a much larger support staff in non-medical occupations, mainly in the running of hospitals, an area in which dentistry has a very minor commitment.

Rationing Dental Care

Therefore, while in many ways dentistry stands as the prototype personal health service, with its dominant philosophy of prevention, regular health maintenance and incremental care, the commitment of resources under such a model of service delivery clearly rules out its applicability in the broader health field. Indeed, it is in this respect as well that dentistry highlights both the problems and the special promise of the personal health services since, perhaps more than any other field, it illustrates the gap between practice and precept in the application of non-clinical strategies, especially those founded on the expertise of the social sciences. While the majority of dental educationists strive to produce the perfect technician, and while researchers seek a breakthrough in the biomedical sciences (for a caries vaccine or the like),[10] the current impact of such activities on the oral health of the community is minor compared to the potential gains to be drawn from other strategies.

For example, the immediate potential for increased productivity in the dental surgery is enormous; not only could the capacity of the average dentist be doubled immediately by lengthening the interval between check-ups with no fall-off in the standard of care (Sheiham, 1977: 442), but this capacity could be further doubled by the judicious use of auxiliaries.[11] Furthermore, the employment of preventive workers such as oral hygienists would go far to reduce the necessity for extensive restorative work.[12] Other innovations in the organisation of care and in payment mechanisms have well-established benefits both for access and treatment style.

Finally, legislative strategies in nutrition (Ringen, 1979) and public health (Terris, 1976) provide ample opportunity for advances in prevention. It is in this respect that dentistry illustrates so clearly both the promise and the special problems of the personal health services in an era when the professional is increasingly being called upon to consider alternatives to traditional treatment strategies and, in particular, to adopt methods of practice attuned more to controlling the effects of ageing and environmental pressures, rather than the traditional skills of curative medicine.

This question of the rational organisation of services to meet defined human needs is, of course, a very much broader one. With the rapid growth of the service sector, the involvement of the state and rising public expectations, these issues of defining social need, organising strategies of intervention and, above all, allocating resources to fund such initiatives, have become fare more prominent and present novel intellectual problems for which we are poorly prepared by conventional categories of analysis.

While the issues are complex and vary in different service sectors, there are two themes in particular that run through much of the debate on the human services. In the first place, it has become increasingly clear that much of the conventional apparatus of market economics just does not apply in the analysis of those human services where the rationing of resources is expected to follow principles of defined social need rather than the vagaries of market forces.[13] Secondly, it is becoming increasingly evident that the major issue facing the human services is the relationship between those who provide the service, especially the professions, and those who have a right to receive it. What is problematic about this relationship is that the requirements of occupational self-advancement — the 'trade union' functions of those delivering services in the community — may not necessarily coincide with the wider public interest, and it is these 'trade union' functions of protecting and improving occupational interests that so frequently govern decisions about the organisation and delivery of care, in default of any countervailing pressure from the state or from organised consumer groups.[14]

In both these areas — rationing and professional dominance — dentistry illustrates very well the broader questions that face the human services in the future. While oral health problems lend themselves to a preventive and incremental strategy of delivering care, in fact the vast bulk of dental work is strictly reparative, a pattern that is reflected in the dental curriculum and in the dominant philosophy of practice.[15] If we adopt the conventional categories of *laissez-faire* economic theory, with dental care a commodity that is bought and sold in the market place, then clearly the problem of rationing, which must inevitably arise where resources are scarce, is solved by prices — choking off demand — and by a particular pattern of practice, the premature extraction of teeth, that eliminates future demand for professional services. On the other hand, if we assume a public service. mode where the identification of need is assumed to dictate the delivery of care, then, given the treatment philosophy that dominates contemporary dental practice, this would entail a level of resources committed to dentistry that would exhaust the health budget of all but the most affluent nations. Again, some system of rationing is required.

The question of professional dominance is closely related to the issue of rationing dental care since the social mechanisms that have been developed to control and monitor the distribution of services in the community evolved in a period in which dentistry was striving for professional status and was seeking above all else to promote its occupational cause. Therefore, present arrangements and philosophies in the organisation and delivery of care bear the stamp of a particular historical period in which dentistry struggled to achieve professional status. It is the logic of professional advancement, worked out in the very special historical circumstances of early capitalist society, that goes far to explaining the particular character of the problems that contemporary dentistry faces in adjusting to new social mechanisms for controlling and rationing the delivery of dental care. It is in order to appreciate this problem of professional dominance and the public interest that we have first to consider in some detail the evolution of organised dentistry, since much that we need to understand about the question finds its origins in the history of the profession over the last 150 years.

Notes

1. Menzies Campbell, 1958: 82.
2. Ibid.
3. According to Kelsall's 1955-6 study of British university students 28-30 per cent of all students were from working-class homes, but this was true of only 16-20 per cent of medical students and 15-16 per cent of students at dental school (Elliott, 1972: 67). Furthermore, data from the USA on occupational prestige show that as early as 1947 dentistry featured in the top 20 per cent of occupational rankings (Willcocks and Richards, 1971: 131).
4. See Bell (1965; 1973).
5. This was evidently an important factor in the rise of the medical profession

in the nineteenth century. For the case of the general practitioner in the UK, see S. Holloway, 1964: 316. More recently it has been estimated that the growth in income and rising levels of educational attainment over the period 1950-65 accounted for a possible 54 per cent increase in the demand for dental care in the USA (Cole and Cohen, 1971: 39). Similar factors were probably at play in expanding the market for dental services in the nineteenth century.

6. The proportion of the work-force in white-collar employment in the UK is still under 40 per cent (Kumar, 1976: 474).

7. In 1966 37 per cent of all degree-level qualifications were held by individuals working in the educational, medical or dental services (Rosenbaum, 1971: 7).

8. Castles and McKinlay (1979) report a strong inverse relationship between the extent of public welfare provision and voting support for parties of the Right. The analysis was based on data drawn from 19 advanced democratic states.

9. In a national survey of American adults carried out in 1965, only 29 per cent of those interviewed felt that dentists were trained to deal with all disorders of the mouth (O'Shea, 1971b: 23). Dental students also feel that they have this image. In a survey carried out on a sample of dental students by Quarantelli (1961: 1314), 60 per cent believed that the public saw them as having 'only mechanical skills'.

10. It has been estimated that 75 per cent of biomedical research in US medical schools is funded by the National Institute of Health, much of it in crash programmes on cancer and dental caries (Chubin and Studer, 1978: 67-8). Federal funding in the USA for dental research has increased from $1.78 million in 1950 to over $40 million in 1973 (Morris, 1973: 993).

11. In the 1965 American Dental Association (ADA) survey, dentists with four or more auxiliaries were 85 per cent more productive than the average. The average ratio of auxiliaries to dentists at this time was 1.5 (Cole and Cohen, 1971: 32-3). Also, see Lotzkar *et al.*, 1971: 1079; Abramovitz and Berg, 1973.

12. It is estimated that one hygienist could produce a 50 per cent reduction in caries-incidence for 2,000 children, at a fraction of the cost of the fillings that would have to be placed if those cavities were allowed to form (McKendrick, 1971: 224). If account is also taken of the time it takes to train a dentist and the higher salary levels of graduate dentists, the cost: benefit ratio becomes very much more favourable (Sheiham, 1973: 8).

13. This issue has been developed at some length by economists studying the British NHS. See M. Cooper, 1975.

14. Freidson (1970) has coined the term 'professional dominance' to refer to the way in which professions have come to dominate developments in the social organisation of their occupational area of concern.

15. The dominant philosophical position in this regard is the so-called 'restorative philosophy'. For a discussion of this position, see P. Holloway, 1975.

2 THE EMERGENCE OF ORGANISED DENTISTRY

The majority of those occupational features that we now take to be especially characteristic of contemporary dentistry reflect not so much the outcome of some natural logic of organisational development, as the product of the rather unique social and economic circumstances that accompanied the industrialisation of Europe and North America. Before the advent of the market economy and, with it, the growth of the manufacturing sector and the emergence of a relatively affluent urban middle class, the medieval guilds formed the basis for the occupational organisation of the personal service sector. While the accounts are conflicting in some respects, it does seem that the earliest forms of guild organisation in this area were affected by developments in the medieval church. Menzies Campbell (1970: 524), for example, maintains that it was the prohibition of a twelfth-century Pope that stopped priests from carrying out work which involved the shedding of blood, and that this paved the way for the emergence of a specific lay occupation in this area. In a variation on this theme, Gullett (1971: 9) asserts that it was the action of a thirteenth-century Pope, in prohibiting monks from wearing beards, that established shaving as a fashionable practice and led to further occupational specialisation and development. Whatever the truth of the matter, it is clear that guilds were indeed formed in the personal service sector in the thirteenth and fourteenth century and that in time there emerged a broad division of occupational tasks between barber-surgeons who were permitted to extract teeth, bleed, cup, leech and perform minor surgery, apothecaries who dispensed medicaments, and physicians who attended the sick.

Although this very broad division of labour can be detected in contemporary health services, there is less continuity than one might suppose since this early guild structure had first to be dismantled and then reconstructed in order to meet the strains imposed by the rapid social and economic changes of the industrial revolution. By the end of the nineteenth century the creaking structure of guild organisation had succumbed to the enormous stresses imposed on it by the decline of feudal institutions and the emergence of the new industrial order. In its place there had evolved a principle of occupational organisation that owed very much less to the sponsorship and patronage of the state, crown, church or aristocracy, and instead reflected the social require-

29

ments for survival in a world dominated by market forces and a rapidly evolving and proliferating occupational structure.

The Guild Tradition

But while the stamp of market institutions is clearly discernible in the structure of occupational specialisation in the personal service sector, there are nevertheless marked continuities with the earlier guild tradition. In the UK, for example, dentistry emerged under the aegis of the Royal College of Surgeons — direct successor to the original company of barber-surgeons (Menzies Campbell, 1970: 524). To this day the dentist's office is known as a 'surgery' in Britain.[1]

In fact, it was largely because of the weight of precedence and the guild tradition that the earliest developments in the evolution of an autonomous dental profession took place not in any of the major European centres of medical and surgical excellence but in the USA. In France, major intellectual advances had been made in dentistry in the early eighteenth century with the work of Fauchard (Lufkin, 1948: 95) and it was in the Paris hospitals of the early nineteenth century that the first major steps towards a distinctively modern system of medical knowledge were made (Waddington, 1973: 211). In Germany, the spectacular developments in laboratory science of the second half of the nineteenth century laid the basis for modern scientific medicine (Jewson, 1976: 230), and Bismarck's state-initiated health insurance scheme provided an economic impetus for the modern health professions (Pflanz, 1971: 315). England, the first country to industrialise and to develop market institutions, was another centre where, because it led in so many other areas, one might reasonably have expected the early emergence of autonomous dentistry. Yet, while the industrial societies of nineteenth-century Europe provided the essential technical and economic basis for occupational development and diversity in the health area, the all-important social and political conditions for the emergence of an independent dental profession were not present. Instead, organised dentistry emerged as an autonomous force in that society where the hold of traditional feudal structures was least secure: the new settler society of the North American continent.

What the future USA lacked in the scientific and material base for professional development, it more than made up for with a decisive political break with the old order (the War of Independence)[2] and social conditions of great fluidity, unbounded optimism and growing affluence.

This combination of favourable social and political circumstances stimulated innovation and experimentation in many areas, but in particular it produced in the mid-nineteenth century a quite remarkable period of exploration and change in the personal health services. For example, the first national medical association formed in the USA was not the future AMA, but the American Institute for Homeopathy, founded in 1844. The AMA was founded shortly after, in 1847, but at this time it represented only one struggling school of healing practice among several and followed a rival philosophy of treatment — allopathy — that relied heavily on the extensive use of drugs, bleeding and other 'heroic' remedies. In fact, as late as the turn of the century this group, the allopaths, accounted for only a tiny minority of all those employed in healing occupations, drawing largely on the medical researchers and educationists affiliated to the hospitals (Berliner, 1975: 581).

Innovation and change also characterised the development of surgery in the USA during this period. Largely freed from the restrictions which, in Europe, shackled surgery in a subordinate status to medicine, American surgeons were far more daring and adventurous in the operations they attempted than their European counterparts. Historically, developments within surgery have been important in the evolution of dentistry and therefore the international pre-eminence of American surgeons is particularly significant. Doubtless similar conditions of professional freedom existed in the dental field and probably greatly aided the emergence of independent dentistry (Shryock, 1948: 149-52).

It was in these rather fluid social conditions that organised dentistry developed in the American context. Economic factors were also important since in the USA a large and growing affluent middle class allowed practitioners to support themselves on a direct fee-for-service basis and this provided the foundation for the evolution of a stable system of solo practice. In Europe, by contrast, alternative economic relationships were being developed because, unlike the situation in North America, only those practising in the wealthiest areas could support themselves comfortably on direct patient contributions. Hence, sickness insurance was introduced in Germany, and in England, as in other European countries, many medical practitioners were directly employed by Poor Law agencies and friendly societies (W. Rothstein, 1973: 169-70). The existence of a rather unique set of economic conditions, therefore, contributed to the early emergence of independent private practice in the USA. Finally, we have to take account of the pervasive egalitarianism of the Jacksonian Democracy era which, together with the ever-expanding opportunities of the frontier in the West, provided the ideal conditions for entrepreneurial activity, equally in commerce and the personal services.[3]

Therefore, while dentistry evolved under the aegis of medicine in much of continental Europe, in North America dental practitioners had, by the middle of the nineteenth century, already established for themselves a relatively stable sector of the market for personal health services — along with a number of other medical occupations, such as the allopaths, the homeopaths and other groups vying for a place in the personal service sector. Of course, American dentistry owed much to scientific and technical developments in Europe — first, French dentistry, then German scientific medicine — and the state was still to play an important role in establishing a formal occupational monopoly. Apart from this, however, dental practitioners of the New World owed little to the institutions of the old and relied almost entirely on their individual entrepreneurial skills in opening-up and organising the great potential market for dental services.

If the decisive factor in the evolution of dentistry in the USA was the loosening grip of traditional institutions, in Europe, by contrast, there was a far clearer historical and organisational continuity with the guild structure of the Middle Ages. By the end of the eighteenth century the greater medical profession in England, for example, was still very much as it had been since the Middle Ages. In other words, it was still basically an estate system in which each constituent order or estate was a closed, self-governing body with a clearly defined set of functions and a well-established status within a traditional heirarchy. In England there were three such estates, each regulated by a corporate body after the manner of the medieval guilds; in order of precedence they were, the Royal College of Physicians, the Royal College of Surgeons, and the Worthy Company of Apothecaries (S. Holloway, 1966: 107).

In reality this division became blurred as the lines of occupational development followed by physicians, surgeons and apothecaries became increasingly intertwined. A particularly important development in this respect was the evolution of the apothecary into the role of a general practitioner, a process that was largely complete by the middle of the eighteenth century (S. Holloway, 1964: 306). The old division of labour between the physician who diagnosed illness, the surgeon who was permitted to cut into the body, and the apothecary who dispensed, became increasingly blurred in practice, and by 1850 the far more important specialisation of function was that which had evolved between the consultants on the one hand — the Royal Colleges (of Surgeons and Physicians) — and the general practitioner on the other (S. Holloway,

1964: 314). Despite this blurring of function that took place in all but the wealthiest practices, traditional status considerations contrived to maintain the old divisions. In particular, the Royal Colleges feared the incorporation in any unified medical profession of manual and trading elements such as midwifery and pharmacy that were an important part of the general practitioner's work (Waddington, 1977: 12). Therefore, the Medical Registration Act of 1858, which set the seal on the future shape of the profession, represented something of a compromise since, although it recognised the legal equality of the three groups under the General Medical Council, the trio of medieval guild corporations remained, thus retaining the structure of the archaic estate system (Parry and Parry, 1977: 827).

Drawing the Boundaries

It is against the background of this extraordinary longevity and persistence of medieval forms that the eventual emergence of dentistry has to be understood. For example, it was not until the early-seventeenth century that the apothecaries — the dispensers — split from the Company of Grocers, thus distancing the future pharmacist and general practitioner from their trading origins; and it was not until the early-eighteenth century that the surgeons and barbers parted company (B. Hamilton, 1951: 149), a split that again separated an aspirant profession — the surgeons — from its trading origins and that was to be repeated later in a further split, with the departure of the dentists. Although we cannot infer too much from a limited number of historical examples of this sort, it is possible to detect a certain pattern about the way in which the modern medical occupations evolved out of the medieval guild structure. In each of these instances, an aspirant occupational group attempts to break free from the restrictions placed on its activities by the traditional guild framework and, in doing so, bids to establish its claim on a distinct area of work. But, unlike similar developments in North America, the break is never complete and in each case the secessionist groups is constrained to a greater or lesser extent to operate within the bounds set by the guild tradition.

There was a similar pattern in dentistry. By the 1850s some British practitioners wished to emulate the example of medicine — and the precedent set in the USA — by following the classic route of the 'qualifying association', with its insistence on formal educational requirements as a first step towards the ultimate goal of restricting entry and establishing an occupational monopoly.[4] However, as in the case of medicine and the law, there was a considerable gap between the social elite of the profession — who were the main proponents of change — and the vast mass of practitioners.[5] Furthermore, there was the split between those favouring a link with the Royal College of Surgeons — these were the odontologists — and those working for an independent profession along the lines established in the USA. Again, as in the case of the evolution of occupational specialisation within medicine, tradition exerted a decisive influence, the odontologists won the day, and dentistry, although recognised as a distinct occupational entity, remained under the aegis of medicine as a surgical specialty, a position it held for well nigh a century. Therefore, while a professional identity was formed during the same period in which dentistry emerged as an autonomous force in the USA (1830-60), in England the occupation retained a 'marginal' professional status for very much longer, and did not finally win complete autonomy till 1959 (Richards, 1971a: 135).

As in the case of medicine, the evolution and control of the emerging occupational structure within dentistry involved a complex process of reconciling, on the one hand, the requirements for the formal, legislative closure of the market and, on the other, the demands of various interested parties, including those dental practitioners who had been trained under the apprenticeship system, as well as a number of closely allied occupational groups such as denturists, dental nurses and hygienists, and, of course, the established and dominant presence in the health sector, the medical profession itself.

The emergence of the occupational hierarchy in dentistry has as its closest parallel in medicine the progress of the apothecaries from trading to professional status (Richards, 1971b: 6; Kronus, 1976: 16-17). In the case of the apothecaries, the process was in the first instance prompted by a shift in the market for medical services; because the physicians were unable, and largely unwilling, to extend their services beyond the aristocracy and the wealthy urban elite, the apothecaries in the seventeenth century found themselves increasingly under pressure to extend their activities into the practice of medicine itself (B. Hamilton, 1951: 141). Once the precedent had been established, the apothecaries sought to entrench their new functions under the protection of the law, a goal that was secured in England by the so-called Rose case of 1703 (B. Hamilton, 1951: 163). In so doing, the group did not relinquish its traditional functions. Finally, once legal recognition of these new functions had been secured, the now-emergent general practitioner sought to redraw the functional boundaries in such a way as to re-establish the old distinction between the subordinate tasks of dispensing and handling drugs — the functions originally of the apothecary, but now delegated to the chemist or pharmacist — and the dominant function of diagnosis and treatment that was now the monopoly of the newly-constituted medical profession.

In dentistry the process of occupational development has followed a similar path, though the scope for manoeuvre is very much more limited than in medicine because of the more restricted range of occupational skills required in oral care. In fact, given the rather limited room for occupational diversity and specialisation, dentistry has witnessed a quite remarkable variety of groups vying for a place in the market. On the face of it, the history of the emerging occupational structure in dentistry reflects as great a diversity and fluidity as the comparable process in medicine. For example, was the all-important boundary of professional status to be drawn, as the stomatologists advocated, between those with medical qualifications and those without, thus excluding practitioners trained under the apprenticeship system (an issue that greatly divided the International Dental Federation in the 1900s (Ennis, 1967))?[6] Were the apprenticed and unqualified to be permitted to practise as lower-grade professionals as, for example, in Germany (Fereday, 1970) or in Israel (Shuval, 1971)? Finally, the boundary dividing those with a recognised professional monopoly from the rest could be drawn in such a way as to include the unqualified practitioners in a united profession and exclude other groups, which is what occurred in England with the suppression of the 'Derbyshire Dressers' in the 1920s and the opposition to dental hygienists and other auxiliaries in the 1950s.[7]

These issues of occupational development are of no mere academic interest since dentistry, like medicine, continues to exhibit great fluidity. In the USA, for example, it is estimated that, while dentists carried out nearly all their own prosthetic work up to the 1920s, forty years later this work was almost universally put out to dental laboratories (R. Rothstein, 1958: 112), a process that, predictably enough, has been accompanied by struggles over the training and work status of the dental technician. Further dental ancillaries of all sorts — some operating independently like the denturists and New Zealand's school dental nurses — have emerged and provide a contemporary parallel with the fluid occupational conditions that characterised the emergence of organised dentistry as an autonomous profession (De Stefano, 1975: 225-7).

The Profession and the State

The USA, and to a lesser extent England and the settler societies of the British Commonwealth, represent a far clearer and 'purer' case of the classic route to professional status. Typically, in such cases, professionalisation involves an occupational group marking out and capturing, virtually unaided by any other agency, a segment of a highly volatile and fluid market for personal services. Once achieved, it then seeks to obtain legislative sanction for its occupational monopoly of this market, and it is only at this late stage that the state is involved in any way. In many other societies the state has intervened far more actively in the delivery of dental care, especially in funding and even staffing services directed at certain target groups – though it cannot be said that the limited involvement of the state in the dental market in this way has to any significant degree altered what is a more or less well-established pattern in the capitalist West, of an independent profession organising and serving its clientele at will.

Nevertheless, the state has certainly been involved and this has affected the organisation and delivery of care. In England, for example, state involvement in the provision of medical services was limited to the care of paupers and the poverty-stricken in the period up to 1911. That year the National Health Insurance Act was passed and from that date there was a gradual extension of the principle of social insurance and state involvement in health care until a comprehensive scheme was introduced with the advent of the NHS in 1948 (Gill, 1971: 342). A state commitment in public health was also slow in coming. It required major national upheavals, such as the cholera epidemic of 1832, the Boer War and the First World War to bring the cause of public health into the political arena (Dodd, 1968: 78-82). It was against the backdrop of such events, together with the voluntary efforts of private dentists, that dentistry finally entered the realm of state concern, initially in the School Health Service and under the National Health Insurance legislation, and eventually in more comprehensive fashion with the NHS. In the rest of the English-speaking world the extent of state involvement has been limited to charity care for the elderly and the poor, together with dental services in the schools.

In contrast to the Anglo-American world, where the profession has come closest to the entrepreneurial ideal, in the continental European countries the state has been involved in dentistry from an early stage: either in the financing of health care, as in Germany (Pflanz, 1971: 315); or in the direct provision of dental services in the schools, as in the

Nordic countries before the First World War (Burt, 1974: 117); or in the direct provision of the full range of dental services, as in many East European countries since the Second World War. Although the state has been heavily involved in these countries, it is still not clear in what way, apart from finance, this has altered the dominant pattern of dental practice characteristic of the advanced industrial societies.

With few exceptions, the countries of the developing world have presented conditions far-removed from the entrepreneurial ideal because the health professions have rarely been favoured with the economic circumstances that would permit them to build up and sustain a market for their services independently of the state (T. Johnson, 1973: 287-90). Whilst many of the symbols of independent professionalism exist in these societies, in most cases the delivery of personal services is subservient to state control.[8] In the area of dentistry this can be seen in the ready adoption by a number of Third World countries of the New Zealand-style school dental nurse, usually to the great discomfort of established professional interests (Burt, 1974: 125). Much the same pattern is reflected in the treatment of traditional 'healers' in African countries; the state has seldom, if ever, sought to outlaw such groups, usually preferring, despite opposition from 'modern' professionals, to confer legal status or, at the very least, to extend informal recognition (Dunlop, 1975: 583-5).

The early involvement of the state in the provision of health services in these countries is likely to lead to quite different conditions for the development of professional forms, than has been the historical experience of Western Europe and North America. In fact, even in the advanced industrial societies the involvement of the state has modified the traditional course of development in occupational specialisation. While, historically, the medical profession has controlled very closely the emergence of new ancillary groups, there is some evidence, in Britain at least, that state-funding and concern has contributed to the growth of para-medical groups and fostered their independence (Armstrong, 1976: 162).

The Professional Ideal

Despite the evidence of state participation — at a minimal level in the legal recognition of the profession, and a higher level for financing and providing care and sponsoring auxiliaries[9] — the predominant pattern in the capitalist societies of the West has been the development of an auto-

nomous occupational group free to organise and service a well-defined
sector of the personal service market. Unlike medicine, where specialisation, group practice and the dominance of the hospital have all contributed to the erosion of the entrepreneurial ideal, dentistry still retains
much the same pattern of market organisation as it did in the nineteenth
century, though this is probably more true of the USA, where over two-
thirds of active dentists are in exclusively solo practice (Schonfeld,
1970: 84). Dentistry is still at the stage where the individual practitioner
can offer the client a full range of services that might reasonably be required, excepting certain specialist skills such as orthodontics. Apart
from the range of services which the individual practitioner can provide,
a further factor that reinforces this self-sufficiency is the type of equipment used. The dental chair and accompanying unit are used so inten-
sively in dental practice that they cannot easily be shared; the remainder
of the dentist's equipment is not expensive and therefore provides no
incentive for sharing costs with others (Young and Smith, 1972: 240).
With over three-quarters of non-salaried dentists in the USA in solo
practice, dentistry in North America, and to a lesser extent elsewhere,
remains closest to the nineteenth-century ideal of the 'free' profession
(O'Shea, 1971b: 16).

As in the case of other professions with entrepreneurial origins, e.g.
medicine and law, the special circumstances of the 'free' profession in
dentistry — delivering personal services in an entrepreneurial setting —
have provided fertile soil for the development of a characteristically individualistic occupational philosophy that has much in common with the
ideologies of other small entrepreneurs, though differing from the small
businessman, shopkeeper or farmer in the more obviously upper-middle-
class trappings of professional status.[10] Dentistry, more than most other
professions, still retains a work setting that reinforces the spirit of the
personal service entrepreneur. For other groups this spirit of the 'free'
profession is more or less constantly contradicted by the conditions of
work; in particular, this is a function of the growing complexity and
interdependence of work relationships with colleagues, with allied professions and with administrative and auxiliary staff.[11]

Nevertheless, in all these occupations elements of a common professional ideal can be found and at the heart of this ideal is the claim to a
special autonomy in the exercise of the practitioner's art. More than a
craftsman who takes a pride in his work and may justifiably claim a
particular expertise in his field, the professional lays claim to a special
form of judgement that represents the wisdom acquired after years of
formal learning and practical experience.[12] It is argued, therefore, that,

because of the unique and personal character of this form of judgement, it is more or less impervious to external review. This doctrine probably has most force in medicine because of the very personal and private nature of the consulting relationship, but its principal elements are to be found in all professions. Allied to this belief in the special nature of professional judgement is the claim made regarding the inviolable nature of the client-practitioner relationship. In part the special nature of the consulting relationship is merely a reflection of the conditions the professional requires for the exercise of his art; but also the notion is inspired from the nature of the personal service relationship and the direct economic transaction between consumer and provider.

The significance of these ideals is not so much for the guide that they may give to the everyday routines of professional practice, as in the broader symbolic function that they serve in underlining and justifying the necessity for practitioner autonomy and client trust, two central beliefs that find their clearest expression in medicine in the doctrines of 'clinical autonomy' and the special nature of the client-practitioner relationship. In part, such beliefs and values represent the special economic circumstances of the independent profession, reflecting the need to celebrate and justify the special independence of a practitioner competing in the market for personal services.

The idea of a set of beliefs, organised about key occupational interests, is referred to by Barbara Wootton, for example, as the 'ideology' of modern casework in the social work profession (Halmos, 1969: 143). But there are other symbolic and ideological functions served by such philosophies: the need to present the work of the profession to other groups in the community in a favourable light, the need to compete for attention and resources, and the need also to make sense of the nature of the professional task and the recurrent work problems it presents (Elliott, 1973: 211).

The sometimes complex relationship between occupational philosophies and broader social circumstances is well-illustrated in the case of medicine. Before medicine became fully organised as a profession, in the eighteenth century, the relationship between client and practitioner in England was heavily weighted in the client's favour since, apart from the ministrations of the apothecary among the poor, the usual pattern of practice was that of the attendant physician waiting upon a wealthy, aristocratic patron on whose favours and good pleasure he depended for his livelihood. As a consequence of this client-serving relationship, the gentry and aristocracy of eighteenth-century England did much to control not only the consultative relationship but also the entire course of medical innovation and development (Jewson, 1974: 382-3).

The systems of diagnosis and disease-classification developed by physicians in this period were based on concepts of illness with which it was felt the upper-class patient and patron could identify. Characteristically, these systems emphasised the unique, if not idiosyncratic, nature of each individual client's health problems and highlighted the particular aptness of the system of diagnosis and therapy espoused by the attendant physician. By emphasising the more unusual and distinctive aspects of their therapeutic systems, individual practitioners, like latterday psychotherapy cult leaders, sought to attract personal followings among the gentry and aristocracy; at the same time, by stressing the uniqueness of each individual patient's health problems, they sought to justify the necessity for their personal ministrations and for the collection of fees levied for their attendance.

According to Jewson, therefore, the state of medical knowledge in the eighteenth century can be related in quite a precise manner to the social conditions prevailing at the time. The greatest obstacle to any advance in medical knowledge was the intensely individualistic and competitive conditions of practice. Innovation was either jealously guarded as a trade secret and used to further the cause of the individual practitioner or, if revealed, ran the risk of being ridiculed by other practitioners anxious to protect their followings against defection. It was only with a shift in the balance of the consulting relationship from client control exerted by a patron to professional loyalty owed to colleagues that medicine was able to reconcile the individualism of private practice with the co-operation required for advances in medical knowledge. This was only possible once it was the broader profession, not the individual client, that benefited from innovation and judged its worth on the more widely recognised standards of scientific research. A crucial development in this respect was the emergence in the early nineteenth century of systems of medical ethics — more correctly termed medical etiquette — the purpose of which was to regulate the relationships between practitioners, once the rules of patronage had been superseded by the loyalties of professional allegiance.[13]

At the core of the professional ideal, therefore, is the necessity to preserve the individualism and autonomy of the practitioner, while at the same time maintaining some professional unity by restricting direct or overt competition; while the individualistic practice of the eighteenth-century professional gentleman is preserved, his dependence on his clients is curtailed by restricting the degree of competition among colleagues and by emphasising broader professional loyalties. Like the

advent of 'combinations' or trade unions in the occupational organisation of the nineteenth-century working class, the route to professional
status represents an attempt to control excessive, and ultimately self-
destructive, individual competition in the collective interest of organising
and managing an otherwise volatile and unpredictable market (Klegon,
1978; Gyarmati, 1975).

While the clearest expressions of the professional ideal have tended
to come at crucial political junctures (such as the struggle for licensure
or in public debate about organisation, financing and the role of the
state), [14] these more strictly economic and political dimensions of professionalism – the ideology of professional groups – are closely
associated with what one might call a philosophy of practice, i.e. a way
of viewing and organising beliefs and values about the work of the profession. At the broadest and most general level this means that we would
expect to find that the philosophy of practice, the way of thinking
about an area of professional concern such as illness, is affected to a
greater or lesser extent by the broader social circumstances of the profession; so, corresponding to the relationship between rich client/patron
and medical attendant in the eighteenth century we find a characteristic
philosophy of practice, an identifiable view of illness and the task of
medicine that rests in comfortable symbiosis with the social position of
the profession (Armstrong, 1979: 1). The influence of such broad social
circumstances can only define very general intellectual tendencies since,
within these very widely defined conceptual boundaries, there may be
various specific treatment philosophies that reflect the different treatment options open to the practitioner. Leaving aside, for the time being,
these more specific treatment styles, it is clear that the very broad trends
of development in the health professions have been largely shaped by a
quite specific set of historical circumstances. In particular, because the
doctrines of the major health professions were developed in an era in
which the quest for market security was paramount, there has rarely
been room within prevailing philosophies of practice for treatment
strategies, clinical concepts and forms of professional intervention that
do not involve the one-to-one relationship between client and practitioner.

In other words, where the paramount consideration is building up a
stable sector of the market for personal services, preventive and collective strategies of intervention, strategies that do not involve the direct
intercession of the professional, will tend to be neglected. This is probably an overstatement since it is of the very nature of healing professions like dentistry and medicine to highlight the central importance

of the consulting relationship between client and practitioner. They would not be healing occupations if they saw the world otherwise. Nevertheless, the question still remains as to why it is that the philosophies of such healing occupations have come to dominate the entire intellectual orientation of the health field, and the answer must surely rest with the very special historical circumstances in which the major health occupations took on their present form.

The Personal Service Ethic

The prevailing concepts of professional practice in the health area, therefore, probably owe something both to the nineteenth-century entrepreneurial ideal and to the nature of the social functions of the 'healer'. This intellectual tradition would be significant, but of limited importance, if the history of the rise of the medical and dental professions was merely a chronicle of the way in which certain occupational groups have come to allocate among themselves various sectors of the personal service market. But the history of the modern health professions is very much more than this, since it is also a record of the way in which certain personal service occupations have come to dominate not just a section of the market but an entire occupational structure; and with that domination there has emerged a more or less complete monopoly of intellectual developments — to the extent that our concepts and ways of thinking about a certain area of human concern and our notions of how best to intervene in that area are almost entirely fashioned by the mentality of the personal service professional. The medical profession, for example, has not only successfully marked out an area for the exercise of clinical skills, which is what we would expect of a healing occupation, but it has also come to dominate the tasks of health promotion and health maintenance in general and to shape our thinking about strategies of health intervention. Much the same could be said of the dental profession. Although dentistry is associated with a much more limited area of social concern — oral health — the consequences of the intellectual domination of a single occupation are no less far-reaching than they are in the case of medicine.

The proposition that powerful social groups will shape intellectual developments in their area of interest seems plausible enough. One does not have to be an uncritical advocate of Illich's (1977) notion of 'the disabling professions' to see that certain occupational groups make it their business to advance their technical expertise and, in so doing, quickly outdistance and supersede the folk-knowledge of the general public. Nor is it necessarily the case that the professions exert a completely uniform intellectual influence, since they themselves can be quite diverse groupings subject to a range of outside influences (Bridgstock, 1976: 311). Social class, for example, has historically had quite an important effect on the development of treatment philosophies in the health professions. While the physicians and surgeons of early-nineteenth-century England served the gentry, the surgeon-apothecaries worked in those areas that were to become the principal concentrations of the industrial working class, with consequences for the quality of primary care in these regions that is evident even after the advent of the NHS.[15] Similar forces can be seen at play in the delivery of dental services, with quite marked variations in the pattern of dentistry practised in different parts of England; in particular, there is evidence that dentists in the North of England are less preventively-inclined both in their attitudes and in their patterns of treatment, and that this reflects the predominant social-class composition of this region (Craft and Sheiham, 1976: 374-6). Therefore, there are certainly variations within professional concepts of practice, and these variations can be traced – in these examples, at least – to the influence of external social-class factors. Nevertheless, such diversity as does exist tends to occur within rather narrow intellectual bounds and so the impression that we have of a rather monolithic consensus within professional circles is not greatly altered by the evidence on the effects of social class and other external factors.

Of course, there have been periods when alternative strategies of intervention have gained prominence. These have generally coincided with periods of wider social and political change. For example, the French Revolution provided an opportunity for a wide-ranging debate about medicine and its place in society and, for a time, medicine was given a major responsibility for reshaping the social order (Foucault, 1973: 31-44). The publication in England of Edwin Chadwick's *The Sanitary Conditions of the Working Population of Great Britain* (1842), not long followed in North America by Lemuel Shattuck's *Report of the Sanitary Commission of Massachusetts* (1850), stimulated public interest in preventive health (Freymann, 1975: 529-30). In fact, the 1840s saw a considerable amount of activity in North America; for example, the Popular Health Movement with its emphasis on lay participation, and Thomsonianism with its stress on self-reliance, prevention and the treatment of the whole person (Kelman, 1975: 638). At about the same period in the USA there was considerable interest shown in nutrition and the effects of diet. At a national meeting of dental practitioners in 1864, for example, there were comments made about the trend towards the excessive refinement of flour and about sweet-eating among the young (McCluggage, 1959: 152-3). Perhaps the most startling challenge to the conventional treatment philosophy in American dentistry was the rise of the oral hygiene movement which advocated the dental examination of all children, the establishment of clinics for treatment and research, and a mass health education campaign. In 1911, as a consequence of the efforts of the National Dental Association's Oral Hygiene Committee, 3,200 dentists assembled in what was at that time the largest meeting of its kind (Dunning, 1970: 43).

Apart from such unusual occasions, it has generally been the clinician's concept of dental practice that has dominated the deployment of resources and that has also tended to govern our ways of thinking about the problems of oral health in society.[16] Indeed, if there is a logic or rationale to what one might call 'the social organisation' of contemporary dentistry — its internal structure and its intermeshing with other groups and institutions in society — then it must assuredly reflect the grafting of the expertise of modern clinical science onto a flourishing entrepreneurial tradition. Almost the entire enterprise of dentistry is geared to the delivery of highly sophisticated personal services in a practice-setting that has changed little since the nineteenth century.

Notes

1. This also applies to the general practitioner, who is descended from the surgeon-apothecaries of the early-nineteenth century (Tudor Hart, 1972: 351).
2. Berlant (1975: 302) argues that the decisive break with the past in both the USA and England was promoted by important political developments that prepared the ground for the establishment of a professional monopoly.
3. McCluggage (1959: 40) tells the story from these early days of the ex-barkeep who left for the West with a drove of horses and six weeks later reported himself a dentist. Although probably apocryphal, the story gives some idea of the fluid and open character of the dental profession at this time.
4. Qualifying associations were the classic method of mounting the reform of the traditional professional organisations inherited from the medieval guild structure. They introduced internal democracy, greater participation by the membership, and promoted educational facilities and higher educational standards. The first of these associations was the Institute of Civil Engineers founded in 1818. The growth of qualifying associations was particularly rapid in Britain in the 1880s (Millerson, 1964).
5. Much the same conflicts, with origins in traditional occupational differences between lower status general practitioners and the 'gentlemen' of higher social standing, characterised the legal profession in the nineteenth century, as reflected

in the bitter disputes between attorneys and solicitors on the one hand and the barristers on the other (Richards, 1968: 141). This was a general pattern in the traditional professions since these were dominated by a leisured and classically-educated elite who felt threatened by reform movements from below (Roth, 1974: 18).

6. In the USA the Stomatological Movement was largely an attempt by a small, elite group of dentists to raise the scientific status of the profession and break with the tradition of mechanical dentistry (Blaugh, 1935: 1860-1). In Western Europe the model of stomatology has been followed in Italy, Spain, Portugal, Austria and Germany, and to a lesser extent in France and Belgium (Freihofer, 1964). In the Soviet Union (USSR), university chairs of odontology were renamed chairs of stomatology, making dentistry a specialty of medicine. A number of other socialist countries have followed the Soviet model, including Bulgaria, China and Cuba (Ivashchenko, 1970: 511; Vutov, 1969: 525); otherwise Eastern Europe follows the model of dentistry.

7. The Dentist's Bill, which was to accord final independence to the dental profession, was delayed for some time while bargaining continued between the profession and the government over the future of auxiliaries (Editorial, 1974: 371).

8. For an instance of this see Jeffery's (1977) discussion of the case of the Indian medical profession.

9. For a contrary view on the supposed 'sponsorship' of the state, see Eaton and Webb (1979).

10. Klegon (1978: 264) argues that many of the distinctive features of the professions are more properly understood as aspects of upper middle-class life-style, rather than characteristics somehow inherent in this form of occupational organisation. The development of professions is seen here in the special historical context of early capitalist society, with the profession viewed as the middle-class equivalent of the working-class trade union or craft organisation; hence, higher education and university training are the middle-class equivalent of the working-class apprenticeship.

11. Although it is difficult to provide precise information on the relationship between changing conditions of work and broader ideological horizons, there is some evidence from the USA that contrasting organisational settings in medical practice are in fact associated with different social and political attitudes. Goldman's (1974) study of Yale medical graduates and students showed that those in solo practice were politically more conservative than those working in group settings — as were general practitioners also — and held more conservative views about the organisation and delivery of medical care.

12. Medical knowledge represents a special balance of science and clinical experience which, Armstrong (1977: 599-600) argues, has now been upset by the advent of the controlled clinical trial, since this opens up areas of clinical practice to the possibility of evaluation. The early nineteenth-century method of clinical observation (the sixth sense of the experienced clinician), provided a basis for clinical autonomy, a dominant position in the patient-practitioner relationship and a hierarchical authority system based on seniority.

13. Paul Revere (1970: 20), a pseudonymous commentator on contemporary American dentistry, makes this same point in relation to the ADAs code of ethics which, he argues, is defined more in terms of the behaviour of dentists towards each other than their dealings with members of the public.

14. A good example of the attempt to invest the interests of the profession with wider social meaning and to link these interests to broader values is the comment of the President of the ADA, countering moves towards compulsory health insurance in 1946: 'This legislation is a threat to the American way of life. Our States' rights, our personal freedom, the sacred human relationship that has always

existed between professional men and their patients is being threatened'
(McCluggage, 1959: 421).

15. A study in the early 1950s into general practice in Britain found that medical
practitioners in rural and industrial settings had slipped into practice routines that
were the minimum acceptable to their clientele (Elliott, 1972: 117).

16. Nor is this restricted to the capitalist societies. For example, the ratio of
physicians to other health personnel in the USSR is now 1:3, as against 1:10 in the
USA, suggesting a strong treatment orientation. There is also in the USSR a growing emphasis on the biomedical sciences in medical education (J. Cooper, 1972:
723-4). The Canadian Lalonde Report provides data on health expenditure that
may give some more precise indication of the treatment-orientation of contemporary health care systems. Of a total health budget of $244.3 million in 1973-4,
just over 3 per cent was spent on environmental and life-style interventions. The
great bulk — over 90 per cent — went to the organisation and delivery of health
care services (Lalonde, 1974: 52).

3 THE SOCIAL ORGANISATION OF DENTAL CARE

An Emerging Manpower Structure

The history of professionalisation in both medicine and dentistry has been largely a story of the successful attempts of an occupational group to secure its place in an expanding and fluid market, to stabilise and organise that market and then to control the subsequent evolution of its manpower structure. In fact, the very process of organising the market involves the shaping of occupational development; in part this reflects a response to the forces of market demand, but also it is dictated by the manoeuvrings for occupational advancement and supremacy. To take the case of medicine, for example, it is possible to identify a clearly discernible cycle of occupational development; in the first instance, a phase of market expansion associated with considerable occupational diversification; then a stage of intense competition among the different occupational groups vying for a dominant position in the expanding market for medical services; finally, legislative intervention freezes the market and establishes a new pattern of occupational monopoly, giving the now familiar hierarchy of consultant, general practitioner and dispensing pharmacist (Kronus, 1976).

The critical factors in such a process of occupational evolution were:

(1) an established presence in the market, something that worked in favour of the general practitioners who, by the 1830s, provided about 90 per cent of all personal medical services in England (Waddington, 1975: 43) and who were therefore a force in medicine that could not be ignored;
(2) a reasonably large membership, but not one that was so large as to flood the market with practitioners;
(3) some pretensions to educational attainment in order to legitimise the claims for an exclusive occupational domain;
(4) the elimination or subordination of potential competitors and the establishment of an occupational supremacy.

It was this last factor — the potential conflict among competing healing and other service occupations — that was probably one of the most

important issues that had to be resolved in the nineteenth century. Because the medical scene was well stocked with various folk healers, midwives and other practitioners, most of them women, and most of them
providing care for the poor (Ozonoff and Ozonoff, 1975: 302), it became necessary for the emergent medical profession to deprive potential
competitors, such as midwives (Donnison, 1974: 2) and nurses, of much
of their earlier independence and subordinate them to medical control.
In fact, dentistry could well have been viewed in the early-nineteenth
century as just one of many 'specialties' that existed among folk practitioners at this time (Freidson, 1972: 344). This is certainly the implication to be drawn from references made about folk practitioners in the
wake of the legislation of 1815 that gave some legal recognition to the
informal medical practice of apothecaries. A commentator at the time
argued that the Act gave too much independence and tacit recognition
to a range of folk practitioners including 'midwives, herbalists, cuppers,
barbers, electricians, galvanizers, *dentists,* farriers, veterinary surgeons,
village wisemen, and cow-leeches' (B. Hamilton, 1951: 169) (emphasis
added).

In a period in which the medical occupations were fully absorbed in
shaping their own future, the dentist, in the company of a host of other
practitioners, could easily appear as a potential competitor rather than a
future professional colleague. It is therefore probably true to say that
dentistry was in this period regarded more as a competitor, or at least of
subordinate status, since it followed a mode of treatment not entirely
accepted by the dominant medical occupations of the day[1] and so could
not be easily accommodated within the developing occupational
hierarchy.

Nevertheless, dentistry follows much the same pattern of occupational advance as the medical groups, though in a far less elaborated
form because of its more limited area of expertise and skill development.
It is precisely *because* there is so little room for specialisation and skill
development in the dental market that the emergence of a manpower
structure has been heralded by occupational competition. Apart from
anything else, dentistry has had to struggle in the shadow of a powerful
and prestigious medical profession. Aside from the USA where the
'historic rebuff' from medicine in the 1840s (O'Shea, 1971b: 20) meant
merely that dentistry was forced into a vigorous self-reliance, the prox-
imity of medicine in most other countries has delayed the emergence of
an autonomous dental profession. But while the formal recognition of
professional status may have been delayed, the cycle of market expansion and occupational diversity, followed by competition and market

closure, has proceeded in microcosm *within* dentistry, in parallel with attempts to resolve *external* boundary problems with medicine.

As in medicine, where an established claim to a share of the market was important, it was necessary, in England at least, to demonstrate a reasonable ability to provide dental services on a national basis before parliament was willing to grant an exclusive monopoly (Richards, 1971b: 8). A stream of technological innovations from the 1840s onwards (Gies, 1926: 36-7) — anaesthesia, amalgam-filling, vulcanite dentures, the drill, the operating chair, the X-ray — all gave legislators and the public an impression of technical advance and scientific competence.

The only problem that remained, as in the case of medicine, was the existence of potential competitors in the form of lesser-trained female auxiliaries developed in a number of countries to work in the schools — hygienists in the USA (Gies, 1926: 75-8), dental dressers in England (Larkin, 1978: 8), school dentists in Scandinavia (Burt, 1974: 117) and school dental nurses in New Zealand. While in England and the USA these initiatives in the further evolution of the dental manpower structure were either actively suppressed or at least discouraged,[2] in Scandinavia the school dentists were accepted into organised dentistry as professional equals — which probably accounts for the high proportion of female dentists in these countries to this day — and in New Zealand, rather anomalously, the school dental nurse developed as an independently operating auxiliary, a school dentist but one who was not accepted within the established dental profession.

The growth in the number and size of such ancillary groups has been rapid over the last thirty years; for example, the proportion of graduates in the health services has halved, as the percentage of lesser-trained support staff has doubled over the same period. This applies equally to dentistry as it does to medicine, optometry and pharmacy (Adams and Fraser, 1976: 9). More specifically, rapid growth has taken place in the amount of work carried out by dental laboratories and, while the profession has been successful in most cases in keeping control of this process — for example, the success in the USA in making mail-order dentures illegal (R. Rothstein, 1958: XXII) — direct access to the public by denturists is now permitted in Tasmania, Denmark, certain Canadian provinces (Allred, 1977: 8) and, most recently, in the state of Oregon.

In general, the policy of the profession has been to bring already existing auxiliary groups under its direct control and, where this has been possible, to draw the benefits of their productivity by increasing the number of auxiliary workers under the control of the dentist and by forcing down the price of such services to the dentist with limitations on auxiliary training.[3] Where the direct control of such workers has not been possible, the policy of the profession has been to try to force up their prices and restrict their availability.[4]

The great expansion in the number of auxiliaries and the increasing involvement of the state in the financing of dental care has prompted at least one commentator to advocate the alternative manpower model of stomatology (De Stefano, 1975: 227). Under this structure the hierarchy that is implicit in the development and deployment of auxiliaries is more accurately reflected in the formal division of labour. In many of the socialist countries, for example, a medically trained professional – the stomatologist – carries out the initial diagnosis together with any of the more complex clinical procedures, but the bulk of the routine dental work is undertaken by a dentist aided by various auxiliaries.

In a sense it could be said that the manpower structures of stomatology and dentistry are not really all that different. With the growth of specialisation in North America and Western Europe, and a broader concern among dentists with oral condition rather than just dentition, a hierarchy is emerging that is much like that characteristic of stomatology: a small central core of the more highly trained and a much larger group of general practitioners, both groups supported by a rapidly expanding auxiliary staff. The important difference remains, however, that the general practitioner lays claim to diagnostic skills and does not acknowledge any supervision from the specialist. Nevertheless, as in the case of the medical profession before it, and as in the early days of occupational licensure, a dual process of upgrading skills (specialisation) and delegating skills is taking place, a process which, as before, follows a complex interplay of market expansion, technological advance and growing occupational diversity.

Sources of Diversity

This process of growing occupational diversity can be followed within the boundaries of the profession. Quite diverse ideological and political tendencies may emerge, as has been documented in the case of the American medical profession where, in a recent analysis of medical publications, it was possible to identify three quite distinct and consistent ideologies reflecting traditionalist, liberal and radical schools of thought in modern medicine (Harrington, 1975: 913). Apart from the impact of occupational diversity on such ideological developments, it is usually also possible to detect the influence on the emergence of informal groupings in the profession of social factors, such as the ethnic background or social class of practitioners, their educational background, shared professional standards and position in the market for medical services (Bridgstock, 1976: 311).

The effects of the market are to be seen more clearly, of course, in free enterprise systems, like the USA. Freidson argues, for example, that a solo fee-for-service system is inherently unstable because of the necessity to cultivate clients in order to retain their custom and because of the constant possibility, despite such attentions, that practitioners will lose clients to their colleagues (Freidson, 1972: 346). One way in which practitioners can reduce this dependence on clients and on the forces of the market is to enforce an artificial scarcity of supply that maintains services in high demand. Another way is to increase the security of relationships with professional colleagues; in the first instance by making arrangements on an informal basis to cover for holidays and other contingencies, but, further than this, by making more formal arrangements to share facilities and expenses until, at their most formal, such arrangements take the shape of a group practice (Freidson, 1960: 377-81).

While there is evidence that such informal arrangements abound in medicine — for example, such loose networks have been found to be crucial in determining the course of individual careers (Hall, 1948; 1949) — it is not at all clear that dentistry is particularly conducive to the formation of such 'colleague-networks', if only because of the very individualistic and self-sufficient nature of dental practice and because of the lack of any wider career path such as is afforded by the hospital community in the case of medicine (Young and Smith, 1972: 242). One study (Wolock and Wellin, 1971) suggests that, far from it being the case that specialists form a dominant group around which networks coalesce, in dentistry specialists may actually have to ingratiate themselves with general practitioners, rather than the reverse. Therefore, it is maintained, specialists do *not* form the nucleus of a central 'inner fraternity'[5] that controls the distribution of career rewards, a fact that is probably mainly due to the paucity of such rewards in an undifferentiated occupation such as dentistry. Because the centre of gravity in dental practice is still the individual office and not some central institution like the hospital, there are probably few career rewards to distribute.

Furthermore, unlike the case of medicine, there has been little evidence in dentistry of any marked ethnic and religious differences between those informal colleague networks that *do* exist, though in the study by Wolock and Wellin (1971) this could possibly have been due to the fact that the research was carried out in a small, and presumably relatively homogeneous, town. In contrast, there is other work in dentistry that does suggest some diversification within the profession along lines of social and occupational differences. Waldman (1971), for example, has shown that specialists tend to be more involved in the official activities of the profession, holding a disproportionate share of the senior positions in the organisation. It is also evident that many associations exist in the American profession organised around differences of religion, race, sex and specialty (O'Shea, 1971b: 17). Such differences may be reflected in contrasting patterns of practice (Shuval, 1970) and in practice location (Montoya *et al.*, 1978).

One reason for the apparent lack of any marked diversity in dentistry is undoubtedly the overwhelming predominance of solo general practice. The relatively limited range of expertise required is also a factor. In medicine, by contrast, historically quite diverse intellectual traditions can be identified and linked to specific developments in the social organisation of the profession and its work (Jewson, 1976). One does not have to go any further than contemporary medicine to identify varying treatment philosophies within the boundaries of the same specialty — for example, surgery (Knafl and Burkett, 1975) and psychiatry (Strauss, 1964) to name but two.

The diversity of organisational settings within medicine, by contrast to dentistry, also contributes to the heterogeneity of the profession. For example, recent research shows that the type of ambulatory care and hospital setting exerts a far greater influence on the quality of care than does formal medical training, an effect that exists quite independently of specialty (Rhee, 1976; 1977). The influence of different methods of remuneration can also be detected in medicine; fee-for-service tends to encourage higher productivity and provides a more personalised form of service, but a salaried system shows advantages on most other criteria such as the comprehensiveness and continuity of care provided, access to services, and impact on health (Boudreau and Rivard, 1976: 61-2). Although from research by Hall on the social organisation of dental practice in Canada, differences in practice characteristics were not specifically related to variations in service outcome (O'Shea, 1971a).

The Institutional Context

If dentistry lacks some of the organisational diversity of medicine, it is still affected in much the same way by wider social, economic and political influences. This is apparent right from the earliest days of organised dentistry which saw a hastening of the progress towards professional status inspired by the emergence, in a hitherto fragmented and captive market, of other powerful groups that appeared to threaten the independence of the profession. This is particularly clear with the emergence of corporate interests in the American market. For example, the invention of vulcanite in the latter half of the nineteenth century opened the way to cheaper and more widely available dentures. It thus expanded the potential demand for dental services. But in another way this development was a rather menacing one for the profession since it meant that a combine, in a virtual monopoly position, could squeeze the dentist between the cost of materials and the price that could reasonably be charged to members of the public. The Goodyear Corporation attempted to do just this in claiming royalty payments in 1864 from dentists for the use of vulcanite. In so claiming its patent rights, Goodyear threatened to undercut the dentist's independence, and the threat was not finally lifted until the patent expired in 1881 (McCluggage, 1959).

Apart from the direct economic pressures of industrial combinations like Goodyear, there was also the threat that, with cheap and easily made dentures, denture-making could itself be industrialised and the skills of the independent, practising dentist dispensed with entirely. In fact, it was in this period that corporate group practices were first formed, employing dentists and providing cheap dentures direct to the public (Schonfeld, 1970: 80-81). These groups advertised and did profitable work and threatened the established dentist, much in the way that the sudden advances in the cost and effectiveness of amalgam-fillings, introduced into the USA by the Crawcour brothers, threatened the livelihood of other practitioners and sparked off the famous 'amalgam war' (McCluggage, 1959: 232).[6]

It was in the latter half of the nineteenth century that the spectacular advances in corporate power took place, especially in the USA; in the years 1898-1904, for example, 236 corporations were formed in the USA with a total capitalisation of $6,000 million (McCluggage, 1959: 232). Faced by such rapid changes in the economic environment – and the potential threats to professional independence that this entailed – and confronted by the growing intensity of occupational competition, the solution of forming a 'combination' or profession was a natural and rational response.

Since this period developments in the economic field have been particularly noteworthy because of the extremely rapid growth of expenditure in health care and the emergence of a substantial manufacturing sector — what one commentator has called 'the medical-industrial complex' (Meyers, 1970: 90). There are a number of reasons for the rapid economic growth in this area. In the first place, the medical area is attractive to commercial interests because it is profitable, because demand is virtually insatiable, and because the market is largely a captive one in which the state frequently acts as the guarantor for profit (McKinlay, 1977: 461). Another reason for growth in health care is the general tendency for the increasing consumption of all manner of goods and services, including 'health', with advances in the standard of living. This tendency is the 'Engel's law' referred to by Michel (1974: 6) and applies to the level of demand for a whole range of more sophisticated goods and services.

Finally, medicine is one area where there has been a marked tendency for rapid and indiscriminate innovation, a tendency that is in part attributable to the efforts of the economic interests involved, but also due to the technological imperative that lies at the base of the modern enterprise of 'scientific medicine' (Fuchs, 1972: 232). *Fortune* estimated the value of manufactured goods in health care in the USA at over $6,000 million in 1967, of which dental goods accounted for $196 million, a little more than the value of a single product range like surgical instruments. At the time of the *Fortune* report, annual growth of the health care manufacturing sector was approximately 10-15 per cent. Although much of this increase may have been due to the introduction of genuinely new product lines and the expansion of existing production, two important features of this expanding market were the rapid obsolescence of new items and a growing trend towards disposable products (Meyers, 1970).

Dentistry, therefore, works within an economic environment that has quite determinate effects on its organisation and the way in which it functions. Apart from the influence of corporate interests — in earlier days regarded as a threat but now accepted with equanimity — there are other interest groups involved in the dental system such as the state and organised consumer groups, and these have tended to be regarded by the profession with some ambivalence. In Germany, for example, the health insurance agencies took it upon themselves to employ dentists to serve communities that would otherwise be without care; by 1930 10 per cent of all German dentists were employed in this way in 200 clinics (Fereday, 1970: 89). Yet, this initiative (which was at one time viewed as a significant contribution to the expansion of dentistry) was later regarded as a threat to the independence of the profession. The service was progressively run down until, by 1970, only ten such clinics remained and the policy of the profession was to oppose their expansion.

A similar suspicion of the role of the state prompted the British Dental Association (BDA) to stay out of the NHS in 1948; within three months, however, 75 per cent of all dental practitioners were enrolled in the service, the majority for reasons of sheer economic survival (Goldberg and Hagin, 1975: 56). The fact is that before the advent of the NHS many dentists struggled to earn a living (Richards, 1971a: 152), but such was the suspicion of the state that the leaders of the profession preferred to stay out of the NHS rather than risk their independence.[7] In the USA, such has been the history of opposition by the medical association to any form of consumer combination — be it state-sponsored or private — that, as late as 1970, seventeen states still had legislation on the statute book prohibiting consumer groups from owning and operating pre-paid payment systems (Faltermeyer, 1970: 127). Suspicion of such third party developments in dentistry is still widespread in the profession in the USA (Douglas, 1971: 631).

Historically, of course, the state was important in securing legislative backing for professional monopoly and closing the market; it has also been important in the attempts made by the profession to regulate the evolution of dental manpower, especially in the control of ancillary groups such as denturists, dental hygienists and other expanded-duty auxiliaries. More recently, however, the role of the state has changed and it now has a more active function in the area of oral health. In part this change in the role of the state is due to its broader functions in the management of the economy, particularly the concern with issues of efficiency and productivity in a period of low economic growth and soaring health costs; also this change is due to the functions that the state exercises in arbitrating among various political constituencies, especially in relation to questions of social justice and the distribution of resources among different social groups.

The two issues are, of course, closely linked. Because the state is forced to arbitrate among the competing, and usually conflicting, demands of different political constituencies, it is drawn ever more deeply into the task of determining the way in which resources are deployed and also into wider issues of inflation, unemployment and the management of the economy. Similarly, the question of economic management rebounds on the political functions of the state. Because there is now considerable doubt about the impact and efficacy of many medical procedures and much investment in the health sector, political questions of equity and equality of access become more, rather than less, important; it now becomes essential to ensure that resources are concentrated on those defects and inequalities in the system that have till now failed to respond to a less specific targetting of health resources (L. Miller, 1978: 432).

Interestingly, dental care is one area where inequalities have been the most persistent, at least in the case of the USA where trend data are available. While the gap in the use of medical services between the poor and the non-poor in the USA has narrowed over a period in which there have been active efforts to relieve the financial burdens of the indigent, in dental care, where no such efforts have been made, the discrepancies in utilisation between the poor and the non-poor remain as marked as they ever were.[8]

The evidence on the maldistribution of dental manpower is strong for both the USA and for England and Wales. Gies (1926), reporting on the North American situation, noted, 50 years ago, the inadequate provision of services for blacks and rural populations. In substance, little has changed since then, with a persistent and gross maldistribution of manpower as, for example, evidenced in research in both Boston (A. Williams *et al.*, 1969) and New York (Wechsler *et al.*, 1972). In England and Wales there is a clear association between the social class 'map' of the country and the distribution of dentists, school dental officers, private practice and the volume of dental treatment (Walker, 1967: 198). The only service item that does not show this association with social class composition is the distribution of consultants; in this case the allocation of resources is very much more under some form of central direction (Cook and Walker, 1967).

Although the maldistribution of professionals is obviously related to the operation of the market where these forces are permitted to operate freely — Tudor Hart's (1971) 'inverse care law' — there are obviously residual problems unrelated to pure market forces, since even the socialist countries are reported to have difficulties in getting enough medical practitioners to work in rural areas (Field, 1975: 455).

Social Class and the State

The state does not operate in any 'neutral' way — were that even possible — because its major function is to respond to, and channel, the influence of various political constituencies. In the health sector, as in social policy generally, the main thrust of legislation and state initiative has largely been worked-out within the context of the overriding balance of power between the principal social classes in the community.

The importance of this social balance of power is central to the under-standing of most social legislation, especially where potentially redistri-butive policies are involved. This is not to say that specific items of legislation are promoted and championed by specific social classes; rather, the details of legislation are determined by concerned interest groups, but these groups operate within an overall political balance struck between the working class and elements of the middle class on the one hand, and the remainder of the middle class and the ruling elite on the other (Wilding and Wilding, 1972).

The impact of this social balance is clearly discernible in the direction and tenor of most social legislation enacted since the Industrial Revolu-tion. In the late nineteenth century social reforms were introduced by conservative governments concerned about the rising social and political potential of the urban working-class. Perhaps the clearest example of this was the introduction of the world's first health insurance system in autocratic Germany, a measure that was specifically designed to antici-pate and, if possible, forestall the rise of a socialist political movement (Freymann, 1975: 528). In the early-twentieth century social security reforms were introduced by liberal governments under pressure from a rising labour movement, and by the end of the First World War, there was a period of further social reform, hastened by the onset of the Great Depression.[9]

In the USA, even though a European-style labour movement has never successfully bid for the popular vote, the social class nature of political conflict over health care, while muted, is still evident enough. Although neither of the major political parties has any firm social class basis (Anderson, 1972: 577-8), it is the issue of the future-financing of health care which has polarised liberals and conservatives; it is also on this issue that historically the labour unions have been most clearly organised for wide-ranging and sweeping social reform (Bowler *et al.*, 1977: 101). In the period from the end of the First World War through the Great Depression to the end of the Second World War — just as much as in the contemporary political scene — the principal antagonists in struggle were the AMA on the one hand, allied with business-oriented national organisations, and, on the other, the national industrial labour unions, allied with liberals and New Dealers.[10]

In dentistry, of course, the scale of social conflict associated with such changes is much lower than it has been in other areas of social re-form, because of the lower social priority of dental care and its limited economic importance (in comparison with medicine). Nevertheless, it is indicative that in the USA, pressure from organised labour has had much to do with placing third party payment for dental care on political agenda, starting with the agreements made in the 1950s between the International Longshoremen and Warehouse Union and the Washington and Californian State Dental Associations (Dressel, 1969: 102).[11] More have followed since.

This is not to suggest that social class factors are the *only* important formative influences on broad, legislative change in the health arena, nor that social class issues are even necessarily the most important factors to be considered in the full range of health policy questions. But if we concede that there is a political constituency to be satisfied on issues of access to health services of all kinds, and if we further allow that this constituency is likely to be composed of those groups and individuals in society who are most socially and economically disadvantaged, then it is logical to expect that political issues of this kind will be articulated most clearly and most forcefully along lines of social class.

Pressures of this sort have typically lead to the greater involvement of the state in the organisation and delivery of health services, either directly in the provision of services, or indirectly through various financial mechanisms that reduce the direct cost of care to the consumer. In those countries where political issues have been more clearly articulated along lines of social class – those with a more 'socialist' tradition – there tends to be a more active state intervention in the health area, including the provision of dental care (Kostlan, 1974: 71-5).

Conclusion

The social organisation of dental care has to be viewed in the context of the rather unique historical circumstances that accompanied the industrialisation of Europe and North America. It was during this period that, under various economic pressures and in competition with other groups of health practitioners vying for a place in the personal service market, dental practitioners organised themselves into a 'combination' or profession, just as many other occupational groups were attempting to do at this time. The dynamics of occupational competition, and trends in the organisation of highly skilled white-collar work, have since resulted in the typical hierarchy of specialist, general practitioner and various ancillary workers that we associate with the occupational organisation of contemporary dentistry.

In its turn, this structure is enmeshed within a web of wider social, political and economic interests. The sugar lobby, and food manufacturing interests generally, attempt to foster a climate of opinion and a professional style of practice that stress the curative and reparative rather than the preventive aspects of dentistry. The dental supply industry is also geared to a high-technology style of professional service that markets products developed for a range of tasks of dental repair and reconstruction. Both blocs of economic interest — food manufacturers and the dental supply industry — operate within broad limits set by the social and cultural environments of advanced industrial societies, i.e. patterns of food consumption, self-care and dental utilisation which control the economic boundaries of dentistry.

The socio-political context is framed by the state and by the actions of broadly based socio-economic groups. While at one time the role of the state in dentistry was merely to set the necessary legislative seal of approval on the attainment of professional status, it has since become far more active in the dental market, both for economic reasons — the management of the economy — and for political reasons, such as the more equitable distribution of professional services. Much of the pressure for growing state intervention has come from those groups that are disadvantaged by the market distribution of goods and services, principally the working class acting through the trade unions and mass political parties. While the form in which these pressures are articulated varies greatly across different countries, its principal outcome has been a greater involvement of the state in the financing and organisation of dental care. Socio-economic conflicts and pressures, therefore, have done much to structure the broader political environment in which organised dentistry has emerged.

Notes

1. In Wardwell's (1972: 250) usage a dentist is a 'limited practitioner' since the service is confined to one part of the human body. But Wardwell also uses the term 'marginal' to refer to a form of therapy that is not acceptable to the medical profession. Dentistry in the early-nineteenth century probably qualifies under both headings.

2. Gies (1926: 78) reports that in 1925 there were 1,750 dental hygienists in the schools in the USA, but this initiative never developed into a full-blown school service. In England, the dental dresser scheme was abolished under pressure from the profession in 1923 (Larkin, 1978: 8).

3. The development of dental laboratory technicians, hygienists and assistants has been kept strictly under professional control (Feldstein, 1977).

4. Where denturists have been able to compete directly with the profession in the supply of dentures to the public, prices have fallen (Feldstein, 1977). In England auxiliaries have, in the first instance, been opposed by the profession and

then, once grudgingly accepted, their numbers and their deployment have been strictly controlled (Manning, 1970: 413; Editorial, 1974: 371).

5. This is not to be confused with the American dental fraternities which probably wield considerable power in dispensing patronage and in controlling key professional jobs. The most powerful of these is probably Delta Sigma Delta founded in 1883 in Ann Arbor (USA), but now with an international network. Key positions in the profession in many English-speaking countries are controlled by members of this group.

6. Lufkin (1948: 205) reports that the so-called amalgam war went so far as to produce prohibitory legislation in the major states in the period 1868-76.

7. This repeated the experience of the general practitioners whose leaders, it seems, were prepared to stay out of the proposed National Health Insurance Act of 1911 because it involved a panel system (Tudor Hart, 1972: 353-4; Parry and Parry, 1977: 828).

8. While there has been an overall increase in the numbers seeing a dentist, and an overall increase in the number of visits made, during the period 1964-73, the differentials remain (Wilson and White, 1977).

9. Sigerist quoted in Navarro (1975: 87).

10. It has been said that the AMA's lobbying efforts against the medicare legislation were probably the costliest ever mounted by the profession (Cordtz, 1970: 132). Cornely (1971: 13) estimates that the AMA spent $2 million on political and legislative activities in 1970.

11. Some American commentaries still have a 'cold war' flavour about them. For example, in the illustrative story used to provide a human interest angle in Young and Striffler (1969: 181) the young dentist, who has recently set-up in the community, has to decide whether the approach from a labour union for a dental plan is 'legitimate' or whether it is a step towards 'socialised dentistry'.

EPIDEMIOLOGY, SOCIAL STRUCTURE AND
THE PUBLIC HEALTH TRADITION

The overwhelming commitment of resources in the field of oral health is to clinical dentistry. This is reflected in the growth of the dental supply industry, which is largely organised around the requirements of clinical practice, and also in the development of a dental manpower structure that has been formed almost exclusively to service the needs of individual client care. Associated with this overwhelming emphasis in the commitment of resources has been the evolution of a set of ideas, concepts and theories about the etiology and appropriate management of oral health problems that is celebrated in a professional mystique about the special nature of the consulting relationship between client and practitioner.

Such developments in occupational structure and in the evolution of professional ideology and philosophy are hardly surprising, given the origins of organised dentistry in the personal service sector. The argument so far seems clear. What *has* to be explained and appreciated is that these ideological and organisational attributes — specifically linked to the requirements of a personal service profession — have come to dominate the entire field of oral health.

The Legacy of Public Health

Much the same observations could be made about medicine, though it has not always been this way, nor has there been great uniformity in this respect across national boundaries. The earliest instances of public health activity in nineteenth-century England were occasioned by certain disastrous health problems of the time — such as the cholera epidemic of 1832 that lead to the founding of the Poor Law Commission (Dodd, 1968: 78) — scattered events which came to be part of a wider intellectual and social movement. Out of these early developments grew notions of etiology and health intervention that stood apart from, and to some extent in opposition to, the traditions of clinical medicine. For example, when the medical practitioners attached to the Poor Law institutions of the 1830s — forerunners of the future medical officers of health — were asked to prescribe treatment and medication for the wretches consigned to the charity of the local authorities, it was clear to most that what these victims of urban squalor required was not any conventional medical therapy but adequate nutritious food and shelter. The duty of the Poor Law Guardians, however, was to reduce the burden of outdoor relief on the rates, not to increase it. Therefore, food and drink could not be accepted as 'treatment', and so this early initiative in preventive health foundered (Gill, 1971: 343).

By the middle of the century, major public health reports had been published both in England and in the USA and these reports led to some important legislative initiatives. However, there failed to develop from these an alternative philosophy of health intervention challenging prevailing notions about the delivery of personal medical services in the community. Instead, rather than providing any philosophical alternative, the sanitary reformers looked to administrative solutions, and in particular to some centralised state machinery for public health. Even these meagre endeavours were to be confounded since there actually never emerged any single national health authority concerned with the expanding role of the state in preventive and curative medicine (Parry and Parry, 1977: 828). Ultimately, for want of a congenial philosophical and organisational environment within the profession itself, prevention became solely the concern of the state. With strong emphasis on sanitary engineering and the dominance of medical education by hospital medicine, preventive activities evolved outside the mainstream of modern medicine (Freymann, 1975: 537). Only in Germany, with the work of Virchow and the Austrian Frank (Freymann, 1975: 528), was there any major philosophical departure from orthodox medical thinking. In this case, however, promising beginnings were soon overshadowed by the other achievements of German science, the spectacular advances in laboratory medicine, which lent their great scientific prestige to the cause of curative medicine in the latter half of the nineteenth century.

Apart from the idea that the state has a responsibility in public health, and aside from the beginnings of such an administrative presence, albeit fragmented and localised, one other legacy of this period was the emergence of certain theoretical and methodological concepts that were to become the central intellectual achievements of the modern discipline of epidemiology in the study of the distribution and determinants of death and ill-health. While the approach has certain continuities with the census tradition of social accounting and the population survey, its development in the late-nineteenth century reflects a significant departure because of the clear association that epidemiological investigations had at the time with the cause of active reform and social intervention.

While the Chadwick and Shattuck reports of the mid-nineteenth century did much to aid public understanding of the potential social basis of health problems and so paved the way for a non-clinical strategy of health intervention (Kelman, 1975: 628), it was John Snow's classic study of a cholera epidemic – *On The Mode of Communication of Cholera*[1] – that provided the scientific justification for legislative action. In a similar way in dentistry, the detective work carried out by McKay on the effects of water fluoridation provided at least the opportunity – if not also the necessity – for legislative initiatives.[2]

Central to the intellectual framework of nineteenth-century epidemiology – and much work in that tradition since then – are the attributes of age, sex and race and, to a lesser extent, social class. The biological trinity of age, sex and race highlights the intellectual origins of the model in a period that witnessed the triumph of Darwin's theory of natural selection and the first spectacular breakthroughs of laboratory medicine. Both Darwinism and bacteriological theory seemed to confirm the essential importance of biological processes across the entire spectrum of scientific endeavour. Even the concept of social class, freshly re-interpreted in specifically sociological terms first by Marx and then by Weber, obtained a biological significance in the theories of the inheritance of talent and of 'the survival of the fittest' developed by eugenicists and Social Darwinists. Therefore, it is not surprising, given this intellectual and social background of epidemiology, and given the traditional focus of dental care and treatment, that thinking about oral health has almost exclusively been within the confines of biological concepts and theories.

Age and 'Social' Age

It is natural that age should be at the heart of any epidemiological model of investigation, both because the maturing of the oral condition is signalled by such clear physiological stages of development and also because of the cumulative and time-dependent nature of the oral diseases. The elderly are one group of special interest and a number of studies have been carried out in this area.[3] Because of the evident frailty of this group, it is natural to seek an explanation for their poor oral condition in the inevitable effects of ageing and gradual physical degeneration. Yet, as both Australian and Norwegian studies show, this generation suffered particular disadvantages and deprivations in their past dental care. In the Sydney sample about 50 per cent of the elderly edentulous patients studied had never had any restorative work carried out whatsoever (Ettinger, 1971: 90), and in the Troms sample two-thirds of those interviewed had never received a filling in their lives (Rise and Helöe, 1978: 8). Therefore, in these two instances at least, it appears that the special circumstances of the elderly may derive just as much from specific social factors – in this case, generational experience – as they do from the physical conditions of old age itself.

To talk, without further qualification, about age differences in oral health, therefore, is to risk entangling and confusing the effects of a number of quite diverse, but still age-related, processes. The conventional understanding of age differences has, of course, been that of physical maturation and ageing. But beyond these interpretations there are two further understandings of the age concept that place almost exclusive emphasis on the role of social factors.

First, there is age as the indicator of generation, reflecting the impact of a unique combination of historical circumstances on the health, values, attitudes and behaviour patterns of the individual. Secondly, age can be a very precise measure of the particular stage that an individual has reached in the social life-cycle, a cycle that stretches from the dependency of infancy through adolescence and family formation to retirement. Such alternative physiological and social interpretations of the age concept considerably complicate the orthodox analyses of epidemiology. We learn, for example, that the increase in caries for most people is very rapid in the pre-school years (Suher and Savara, 1954: 816; Holm, 1975: 228), continuing in this way into the teens, but that it drops in the twenties until a condition of relative stability is reached by the time a person is in their thirties (Jackson, 1961: 91). In the light of what we now know about the social and physical aspects of age, how are we to interpret these results? Are we to implicate basically biological and physiological processes such as the length of exposure to acid attack or even changing qualities of the tooth enamel itself, or are we instead to search for a more sociological explanation – for example, life-cycle changes in responsibility and behaviour, with the irregular eating habits of the teens being followed by the more settled routines of family responsibilities in the adult years?[4]

Similar questions arise in the interpretation of the way in which tooth loss is related to age. A widely quoted figure from an early American study (Pelton *et al.*, 1954: 445) identifies periodontal disease as the primary cause of tooth loss after the age of 35, an interpretation that seems to be consistent with the progressive and irreversible nature of the disease. Yet, in a Swedish study of the pattern of extraction among practising dentists, it is clear that periodontal disease is no more important than caries as a source of tooth loss for any age group, both causes having equal impact at age 50 with about a quarter of the total. In this study at least extraction for prosthetic reasons becomes the dominant cause of tooth loss in middle age (Lundquist, 1967: 303). It is always possible, of course, that these differences reflect major cultural variations. Far more likely an explanation, however, is the different social class composition of the two samples — 70 per cent of the American sample were seamen and coast guards — and the special conditions under which the American study was carried out in the United States Public Health Service (USPHS); by contrast, the Swedish sample was relatively representative of dental users and reflected the interplay of client and practitioner under the normal conditions of commercial private practice. In other words, whatever theory may say about the ageing process and about the expected pattern of oral disease and its impact on treatment, the actual conduct of dental practice is probably more closely governed by economic factors and by the social expectations of both client and dental practitioner.

At the centre of any sociological understanding of age is the appreciation that there are clear patterns in the relationship between age and the culturally established biography or social life-cycle of the individual, and this has important implications for the interpretation of much epidemiological research. For example, 'social' age may be important in affecting the individual's *exposure* to certain risks; among teenagers rough play results in a relatively high rate of accidents to the jaw or teeth (J. Johnson, 1975: 130) and this group is also particularly likely to be eating between-meal snacks (Thomson, 1977: 65). 'Social' age may also affect *access* to care; school-age children provide a natural captive population for the delivery of services in a way that adults do not. Also, because they are dependent and vulnerable, it becomes socially and politically more acceptable to ease the problems of access, especially in those societies where market forces dictate the distribution of services. Like other dependent groups such as the indigent, the aged and the mentally and physically handicapped, children are often regarded as a special case that can be indulged without casting aside the overriding principle of 'user pays'.[5]

'Social' age may also affect social concepts of health since much of the framework that guides individuals in their assessment of personal health is governed by the demands of the key roles they perform in life; hence, with the lower levels of activity that come with retirement, there probably also comes a lowering of expectations of life in general, and of

personal health in particular. Although the elderly consume a disproportionate share of medical resources, much of this is in the form of cust-
odial care, or else is provider-induced, and the indications are that many
complaints among the aged are not taken to the doctor, either because
they are assumed to be an inevitable accompaniment of old age or because it is felt that nothing can be done about them in any case
(Cartwright *et al.,* 1973). It is plausible to assume that with growing
affluence and with higher levels of educational attainment and improving standards of professional care, future generations of the elderly may
well expect more of their oral health and comfort and therefore be far
more demanding of the dental care system than they are at present.

Despite what might reasonably be expected to be a greater objective
need for dental care, the older age groups actually make much less use
of dental services than the young, though how much of this is related to
economic factors and how much to social expectation and generational
experience is not clear. Interestingly, this pattern is the reverse of what
it is in medical care where, as expected from the age distribution of
objective need for medical attention, the very young and the very old go
to the doctor far more frequently than those in the intervening age
groups. In the case of dental care the reverse is the case – the so-called
'inverted U' – with low levels of utilisation among the young and the
old (Wan and Yates, 1975: 145; Andersen *et al.,* 1976: 38). There is
evidence that, in the USA at least, these age differences may be diminishing (Andersen *et al.,* 1976: 39), though the neglect of children's dentistry has a long tradition in that country, going back to the 1930s and
earlier when many dentists would not accept child patients (Burt, 1978:
276).[6] Peak use of dental services – the turning-point in the 'inverted U'
– takes place in the 40-9 age bracket (Moen and Poetsch, 1970: 34).

Sex and Gender

Sex is the other biological variable that, along with age, is routinely
employed in standard epidemiological analyses. The great paradox about
the research evidence in the general health field is that, while women
enjoy a longer life expectancy than men – and have done so since the
eighteenth century – they actually report more symptoms of physical
and mental distress and also make greater use of hospital and primary
care services (Roskies, 1978: 139). Part of the explanation may be
purely biological. It is possible, for example, that women are constitu-
tionally tougher – due to some process of natural selection – and that

they therefore live longer as a consequence. To explain the greater contact with medical services there may also be some biological factor at work, e.g. the requirements of child-bearing. But far more plausible than any explanation couched in terms of genetic and hormonal aspects of women's sexual identity are explanations that relate to the socially and culturally determined aspects of this identity, the so-called gender role.

In a review of the research evidence, Nathanson (1977) argues that the greater longevity of women can be attributed in the main to gender differences in social expectations of behaviour that are deeply engrained in our culture and that mean, in effect, that men are at greater risk than women from death and disease. As far as morbidity and utilisation are concerned — where women, by contrast, seem to be at a disadvantage — Nathanson (1978) argues that the apparent differences between the sexes can be explained by variations in informal understandings about the way in which men and women are expected to cope with physical discomfort, to respond to health survey interviews on the subject and to interact with medical practitioners. Mechanic (1978) in another review of the literature largely concurs with the Nathanson thesis, arguing that women's social obligations give them a greater opportunity for seeking care and being sick and that, further, they may be more prone to report distress since this is culturally more acceptable for women that it is for men. Research by other investigators on women's responses to illness provides some support for this interpretation (Geertson and Gray, 1970: 644; Berkanovic, 1972: 53).

In dentistry the clearest evidence for such sex differences in the response to distress relates to the so-called pain dysfunction syndrome, a condition where pain and discomfort are felt around the jaw and face. While most population surveys report little if any difference between the sexes in the distribution of various sources of facial pain and discomfort (Agerberg and Carlsson, 1973: 335; Helöe and Helöe, 1975: 77), most *utilisation* studies indicate that women are much more likely to seek help for the condition (Franks, 1964: 100; Agerberg and Carlsson, 1972: 597; J. Smith, 1976: 283). On the surface this suggests that, if there really is a psychosomatic element in the pain dysfunction disorder, it relates not to the etiology of the condition but to the way in which men and women cope with the pain and distress accompanying it (Marbach and Lipton, 1978: 635). If *etiology* were also stress-related, we would expect that, as in the case of mental illness (Gove and Herb, 1974; Gove, 1978), higher rates among women could be attributed to the mode and level of stress experienced, rather than to any greater propensity for seeking aid. Weinberg (1977: 204) has argued that the syndrome is not stress-induced but is a tension-relieving mechanism.

Studies of dental utilisation confirm that, as in the case of the pain dysfunction syndrome, women do go to the dentist more often than men (Suchman and Rothman, 1969: 58; Wan and Yates, 1975: 145) and the difference between the sexes in this respect is most marked in the 20-24 age group (Moen and Poetsch, 1970: 36). However, information for the USA on long-term trends in the use of dental services suggests that this discrepancy, such as it is, is decreasing quite rapidly and has declined from a gap of 5 percentage points in 1953 to a difference of only 2 per cent in 1970 (Andersen *et al.*, 1976: 38). In fact, once one has taken into account the relevant variables like age, social class and race, the difference may now be quite insignificant (Andersen *et al.*, 1975: 260).

There may, however, still be an important difference in the style — if not the frequency — of dental utilisation. A review of the literature by Nathanson (1977) supports the view that not only are women less likely to be involved in active risk-taking behaviour, but they are also more likely than men to carry out a range of preventive measures, including a more preventive approach to the use of medical and dental services. This confirms earlier work by Rosenstock (1966: 96), on the use of preventive and detection services, and by Kasl and Cobb (1966: 250) on free health examinations. On specific dental items this pattern shows through very clearly. Teenage girls, for example, are three times less likely than boys to suffer accidental injuries to the teeth and jaws (J. Johnson, 1975: 130), a finding that confirms the picture of risk-avoidance among women. Again on the preventive side, teenage girls are probably also more conscious of the potential ill-effects of sugar, for reasons of personal attractiveness if nothing else (Thomson, 1977: 65).

This more preventive approach is also reflected in the fact that women are much more likely to claim to brush their teeth frequently (Cohen *et al.*, 1967: 230) and tend more often to visit the dentist for preventive reasons (Haefner *et al.*, 1967: 459), both findings which may account for the superior oral cleanliness and periodontal condition of women (USPHS, 1965a; Sheiham, 1969: 120). Paradoxically, for all this apparent show of diligence in self-care and dental visits, women tend to lose their teeth earlier than men and tend to have fewer sound teeth than men of the same age (USPHS 1965b; 1967a; 1967b; Barenthin, 1977: 78). While there could be physiological explanations based on supposed differences between the sexes in their susceptibility to caries (Hewat and Eastcott, 1956: 103-106), an alternative, and more plausible, view is that frequent dental attendance among women means more treatment and therefore fewer sound teeth. Furthermore, for those destined to have their teeth extracted prematurely at some stage, higher utilisa-tion means that this transition to the edentulous state proceeds at a quicker pace than it does among men.[7]

Race and Ethnicity

Race, the third variable in the biological trinity, has found less universal application than age and sex in epidemiological research, but is of parti-cular significance because it lends special emphasis to the social and group nature of what are otherwise too easily interpreted as purely biological differences. In fact, the race concept gives strong intuitive sense to the otherwise rather abstract concept of the social or cultural group, since, whatever else may be said about racial differences, it is undeniable that they can act as very visible boundaries in the formation of distinct social communities.

Although there *is* this potential for the recognition of social and cul-tural factors in the race concept, it nevertheless remains true to say that in earlier applications of the racial category in epidemiological research, it was interpreted in such a way as merely to reinforce the biological assumptions of the day. For example, in early colonial Canada it was widely held that the mixed-bloods had poorer teeth than pure-blood native redskins, not because of their greater contact with European society and its diet, but because of the admixture of European genetic traits that carried with it a higher susceptibility to caries.[8] The theory that there are certain genetically-based racial differences in suscepti-bility to caries is still current among some researchers. In New Zealand, for example, as recently as the 1950s two respected researchers could use what are essentially genetic arguments in accounting for racial differ-ences in oral health (Hewat and Eastcott, 1956: 105-6). A similar hypo-thesis has been tendered more recently in the South African context (Retief *et al.*, 1975: 466).

These examples apart, however, most research involving the analysis of racial factors in oral epidemiology has done much to promote a sociological approach to the interpretation of research data. This is particularly so in the credence that racial differences lend to the concept of the social or cultural group. A researcher who might find it difficult to accept the social reality of differences between socio-economic strata would, by contrast, have little difficulty in grasping the importance of the group concept in interpreting differences between racial categories.

There is, of course, much more than merely a theoretical parallel to socio-economic and race strata. In most industrial societies there is considerable overlap between social class and racial group, with racial minorities in most cases being concentrated in working-class occupations. This means that in many instances, what appears to be a characteristic of minority racial status — such as the low use of dental services — is often better understood in the broader context of social class.

There is evidence for this overlap between race and social class in much that is known about the oral health of minority groups. In what seems to be a common pattern across the full spectrum of the 'diseases of affluence',[9] the upper social strata and dominant white majorities, who were at one time at greater risk from the oral diseases, are now relatively advantaged, though this is more obviously the case for periodontal disease than it is for caries (USPHS, 1965b; 1967a). For the blacks in the USA this transition has been long delayed, suggesting that in some respects their assimilation into the mainstream of the urban working-class is of rather recent origin. Until recently, there was considerable evidence to suggest that black school-age children had a lower caries experience than whites. In more recent studies, however, the advantage seems to have been lost (Bagramian and Russell, 1973: 346; Heifetz *et al.*, 1976: 86), if not in some cases actually reversed (Infante and Russell, 1974: 396).

Explanation for this phenomenon has been sought in changing dietary patterns. Apart from the circumstantial, historical evidence regarding the drift of the American rural blacks to the cities, and by implication their adoption of urbanised life-styles, there is also some concrete survey evidence that blacks may now, if anything, be at a distinct disadvantage in their dietary practices e.g. with a higher consumption of sucrose-containing snacks between meals (Bagramian and Russell, 1973: 346). A similar pattern of assimilation to a Western life-style seems to be evident in South Africa where, until recently, urban black teenagers seemed to have superior dental health to urban whites (Retief *et al.*, 1975: 463-5), but where this advantage is not now evident among pre-school children (Cleaton-Jones *et al.*, 1978: 137). Aside from diet, other aspects of the dental situation of the North American black population suggest a closer assimilation to the conditions of the urban working-class. For example, black adults (USPHS, 1970) and children have a greater backlog of untreated need than whites (Infante and Owen, 1975: 26; Heifetz *et al.*, 1976: 86), which suggests inadequate contact with dental services, as also to some extent does the poorer periodontal condition of blacks of all age groups (Russell and Ayers, 1960: 214).

But the impact of race cannot be reduced entirely to the social and economic conditions of the class structure of advanced industrial societies. The relationship between race and the use of services in the USA is a persistent and continuing one, and it appears to be independent of social class to a significant extent, at least for trend data on medical care utilisation. While the impact of income on the use of medical services has declined over the last 40 years in the USA, the effect of race still remains a powerful one (Bice *et al.*, 1972: 261).

In the case of dental services the difference between the races is, if anything greater than it is in the case of medicine: in the period 1957-60, the proportion visiting the dentist in any given year in the USA was more than twice as high among whites than it was among blacks (39 per cent against 17 per cent); by 1968-70 the rate of visiting among non-whites had increased to 28 per cent — compared to 47 per cent among whites — which suggests that the gap may be narrowing (Andersen and Newman, 1973: 113). Even more striking evidence of the continuing importance of the racial factor over and above the impact of social class is the fact that low-income whites actually see the dentist more frequently than do high-income blacks (Andersen *et al.*, 1975: 261). After taking into account the effects of income, area of residence and education, recent survey information shows that non-whites still have lower levels of utilisation for both medical and dental services (Andersen *et al.*, 1975: 260).

A slightly different picture emerges if our analysis is restricted to those who have successfully entered the dental system. Leaving aside those who have not been to the dentist, the evidence suggests that, once in the system there is every indication that the effect of race is greatly reduced, if not entirely eliminated. For this group, race differences in the *volume* of care received are rather small (Andersen *et al.*, 1976: 40). Despite this apparent similarity in the volume of care received, it is probably still true to say that among those who go to the dentist, differences in the style or pattern of usage still remain; for example, blacks are probably more likely to use public clinics (Moosbruker and Jong, 1969: 727; Leverett and Jong, 1970: 140) and tend to receive emergency dental treatment and extractions rather than preventive and restorative work (Moosbruker and Jong, 1969: 727; Andersen *et al.*, 1975: 261). Again, this style or pattern of usage is very reminiscent of other socially and economically disadvantaged groups in the population.

Apart from the circumstances of inequality, cultural factors are obviously at play in accounting for racial differences in utilisation. This is perhaps most clearly illustrated in research on the way in which people interpret and respond to symptoms. If we take those objective measures of the severity of symptoms and illness that are available, it is clear that blacks approach the medical practitioner or dentist at a more advanced stage and with a more serious condition than do whites, even after taking account of income differences between these two groups. But if we then go to look at more subjective measures — such as respondents' reports of the symptoms that they have experienced — then the position of the two groups is reversed, with blacks reporting fewer symptoms and tending to show less concern about them (Andersen *et al.,* 1975: 186).

What this evidence suggests is that a crucial factor that needs to be considered in explaining racial differences in utilisation is the cultural shaping of the way in which people interpret and respond to symptoms. If we take a uniquely dental symptom — say, toothache — of those reporting this condition in Andersen's study, three-quarters of the whites went on to visit a dentist as against only two-thirds of blacks. Furthermore, this difference between the two racial groups disappeared for those respondents on or below the poverty line, but was greatly enhanced for those on higher incomes (Andersen *et al.,* 1975: 182). In other words, for this condition at least, economic disadvantage is a great equaliser of racial difference, but once material factors become less important — among those on higher incomes who can more readily afford dental care — the impact of different cultural traditions emerges. This finding is confirmed by some research carried out on study populations where the economic barrier has been removed. In Moosbruker and Jong's (1969) study of low-income black and white families in a Boston Head Start programme, the expected racial differences did not emerge. Instead, there were a great number of similarities in patterns of dental care, including recency of last visit, current felt need for dental treatment, making appointments when in need of care and attitudes towards visiting the dentist.

Even where cultural differences *do* exist — for example, in the response to symptoms — they can be seen to be quite closely determined by availability and access to care. For example, Taylor *et al.* (1975), in an analysis of the discrepancy between reported symptoms and actual patterns of medical care use, show that access to a regular source of care is a far more important factor than either income or race. The greatest discrepancy between reported symptoms and actual patterns of medical contact existed for those respondents who had no regular source of care, a result that suggests that the supposed impact of cultural factors must be viewed in the context of the everyday problems of access that people of different racial and social groups face.

This interaction of cultural and situational factors is also illustrated in the pattern of care received among those visiting the dentist. Although there is evidence that blacks are less likely to use preventive and detection services generally (Rosenstock, 1966: 96),[10] it is still true that even among blacks receiving discretionary dental care – that is, care that was sought on their own initiative and without associated symptoms – a far lower proportion receive preventive services than do whites visiting the dentist under exactly the same conditions (Andersen *et al.*, 1975: 182). Moosbruker and Jong (1969: 726) suggest that racial barriers between client and practitioner are important and that part of the explanation of the persistence of these racial differences in the pattern of care is the existence of well-entrenched stereotypes about blacks held by many dentists in the USA. The study by Salber *et al.* (1978) in the American South confirms the impression that such stereotypes may act as a barrier, especially for higher-income blacks who might otherwise be expected to share much the same aspirations for high-quality dental care as the white middle class.

Such cultural and other differences between blacks and whites provide what is probably the most clear-cut community division in the USA, but it is of course by no means the only one. In fact, an emphasis on the more visible attributes of racial difference such as skin colour does much to obscure the importance of other cultural groupings that, like racial groups, have their origins in a common nationality or sense of peoplehood. In the USA there is a multiplicity of ethnic groupings that have their origins in the great waves of migration that have brought many nationalities to the North American continent. It is not surprising, then, that epidemiological and social research in the USA has made full use of the ethnic group concept, though a broad racial (skin colour) classification is also often used. While it is difficult to generalise on the question, it is probably true to say that the black/white distinction is frequently deployed in the expectation that it will cast light on issues of inequality, while the use of ethnic group classifications is more often associated with an emphasis on the impact of cultural factors, usually within an anthropological framework. An example of this approach is the research on the ethnic (and implicitly cultural) differences in the response to symptoms and in the way in which they are presented (Zola, 1966; Segall, 1976).

As far as the utilisation of dental services is concerned, generally speaking Jews have the highest level of dental visiting, followed by Catholics and Protestant whites, then Puerto Ricans and finally blacks (Suchman and Rothman, 1969: 154). Chicanos also use dental services less, and tend to use them less preventively (Garcia and Juarez, 1978: 428). Most of these differences are sufficiently marked to make them worthy of further analysis and it is in order to accommodate variations between cultural groups of this sort that sociologists have tended to use the concept of 'ethnic group' in preference to that of race, if only for the reason that marked ethnic differences may exist within boundaries of the conventional racial classification. More broadly than this, the ethnic group concept gives greater emphasis to the impact of specifically cultural factors in the formation of such groupings, while the race concept still has an echo of an earlier biological and genetic interpretation of group differences.

Social Class

Although there are significant differences between ethnic groups in oral health that can be attributed to cultural variations in diet and self-care (Sheiham and Striffler, 1970; Hankin *et al.*, 1973; Yassin and Low, 1975), many of the differences between blacks and whites in the USA, if not also those between various ethnic groups, can be attributed in the main to the operation of broad socio-economic factors (Andersen *et al.*, 1975: 29).[11] It is here that some of the most marked differences in oral health patterns exist in advanced industrial societies; in this area also the failings of the epidemiological model are most apparent since, while it is evident that behind such socio-economic variations in health and utilisation lie major institutional forces, much of the standard analysis of the evidence on social class remains doggedly individualistic in its interpretation of the data. It is as if Snow, in discovering that the urban poor of nineteenth-century London were using contaminated water supplies, then mounted a campaign to persuade them to use the water supplies in the more affluent parts of town, rather than actually taking steps — as Snow did — to improve the level of sanitation at its source. The emphasis is on individual attributes rather than institutional sources of inequality.

In much the same way contemporary oral epidemiology, forgetting its nineteenth-century origins in the analysis of community structures and group processes, insists on presenting its research in such a way as to play down the impact of institutional settings and wider social forces on the health and service contact of different social groups. Social class cannot be isolated in this way without doing gross injustice to its analytical focus. In fact, social class is a central institutional feature of advanced industrial societies since it reflects the impact of the occupational structure of these societies on the hierarchy of privilege and advantage and on broader cultural and economic circumstances. In tracing the impact of social class we are in effect saying that the workings of many social institutions, including the system of dental care, together with the life-styles and life-chances of different groups, are powerfully shaped by forces that find their source in the occupational and economic structure of industrial society.

Having said this, and having made extravagant claims for the impact of social class, it has also to be admitted that there are some areas where the impact of social class is, at first sight anyway, neither very consistent nor entirely clear-cut. The evidence on the relationship between socio-economic status and oral health presents something of this pattern. Part of the reason for this lack of consistency may lie with the problems of measurement in this area. Socio-economic position has been variously measured by occupation, income and education, using them separately or in combination, and in general the major social strata have been defined in a number of quite diverse ways. Much the same problems of measurement have affected the assessment of oral health; again, different aspects of oral health, various indices, and different components of these indices can all give quite varying results.

Apart from the question of measurement there are other issues. It may just be that social class patterns of oral health are in fact undergoing important long-term changes, in much the same way that change has occurred with the other 'diseases of affluence', and that this is throwing research into disarray. Where at one time, as the term 'disease of affluence' might lead one to expect, it was the upper social strata who were more susceptible to these conditions, it is now the disadvantaged who suffer most from these conditions, as they also do for other health disorders of longer standing, such as the infectious diseases (Blaxter, 1976: 113). Aside from the research difficulties this poses, it is now possible that, if oral health is any guide, the 'diseases of affluence' may well elicit more marked social-class differences than some traditional disorders. In one study (Nikias *et al.,* 1975: 258), where controlled comparison with other health measures was possible, the evidence was that the effects of socio-economic differences were greater for oral health than they were for any other health items.

Despite the problems of measurement and the possible instability of the health picture in the advanced industrial societies, certain patterns do emerge from the research that has been carried out in the area. In the first place, regardless of age group and regardless of research site, higher social strata usually have a lower caries prevalence and, even whether this is so or not and almost regardless of the level of disease, they have less untreated decay and fewer missing teeth, a pattern that probably reflects dental service use rather than diet or self-care.[12] Furthermore, in most, if not all, studies, higher social strata tend to have better scores on measures of periodontal health, at every age level (USPHS, 1965a; 1972; 1974b). While this confirms the favourable health status of the middle class, the mechanisms in this case are probably rather different from those that prevail in the case of the caries measures. An indication of this is the fact that in many studies educational background is more closely associated than income with periodontal health — suggesting that cultural factors, such as self-care, are more important than issues of inequality and problems of service use (Russell and Ayers, 1960: 214; Schonfeld, 1963: 931; Nikias *et al.,* 1977: 201; Plasschaert *et al.,* 1978: 70). It is this mixture of cultural and situational factors that probably also accounts for the delay reported in the presentation of dental conditions for treatment by low-income groups (Andersen *et al.,* 1975: 186).

While the periodontal condition is dependent on personal hygiene and, to a lesser extent, on dental utilisation, the prevalence of caries is influenced mainly by diet, though even here self-care may make a difference. More important than self-care is the impact of dental treatment on the composition, if not the absolute level, of the standard measure of caries prevalence, the so-called DMF index (a simple count of decayed (D), missing (M) and filled (F) teeth). Because the middle class go to the dentist more often, they will probably have more filled and fewer decayed and missing teeth. This higher level of treatment may also influence the absolute level of the DMF index by artificially inflating the F factor over and above normal disease levels.

Concentrating for the time-being on issues of diet, however, there does seem to be some ground for expecting a higher caries level among the lower social strata. For example, at the broadest level, recent information in Britain shows that the diet of the poor contains less fibre, less vitamins and more sugar than the rich (Wilkinson, 1976: 567); a pattern that could be held to account for the greater susceptibility of the poor to a range of health conditions, including dental caries. A number of studies aimed at the specifically cariogenic aspects of diet show that lower-class practices from the infant years onwards tend to be less favourable for future dental health (Goose and Gittus, 1968: 76; Koch and Martinsson, 1970: 63; Pratt, 1971: 289; Roder, 1971: 39; Samuelson *et al.,* 1971: 1371). But the evidence is not entirely consistent, and there is even one study that shows that children from more affluent homes consume more sugar, biscuits and other cariogenic items

(Mansbridge, 1959: 250).[13] Historically sugar was a luxury item and caries an affliction of the wealthy. But the data from contemporary sources suggest that, if anything, the situation is now reversed and that sugar forms a cheap and palatable energy source for low-income households.

If the research on dietary patterns is circumstantial rather than conclusive, information on dental utilisation provides more clear-cut evidence of social class differences. Survey data on dental visiting in the USA indicate that this is one area where socio-economic differentials remain as strong as ever, in contrast to the changing pattern in the use of medical services. While the gap between the poor and the nonpoor in the use of hospital and practitioner services has greatly narrowed, there has been no corresponding closing of the gap in the use of dental services (Wilson and White, 1977: 641). Social class differences do, of course, remain, but the character of these remaining differences has probably altered. Higher rates of utilisation in the middle class are now probably attributable to a more preventive pattern of visiting (Bice *et al.*, 1972: 261), something that is less easy to modify merely by improving access to services and a factor which could go some of the way to explaining the differences that persist in the use of dental services.

It is well-established that the more affluent and the more educated make greater use of a whole range of preventive and detection services, including preventive dental care.[14] This pattern seems to hold at a very general level, since higher-income groups not only use services more preventively but also show a greater propensity to carry out a number of practices that contribute to good health, such as regular eating-habits, exercise, less smoking and drinking, etc. (Breslow, 1972: 352) — a pattern that is also confirmed in the case of personal dental care practices (Kasl and Cobb, 1966: 252; Cohen *et al.*, 1967: 232). Even if we restrict our attention to non-preventive, symptom-related visits, the lower social strata make less use of dental services than the middle class, relative to the level of symptoms they experience (Andersen *et al.*, 1975: 186), a discrepancy that is also found in the case of medical care utilisation (Blaxter, 1976: 120).

Such differences in utilisation have frequently been given a cultural interpretation, and there is evidence for this in the relationship documented for educational level and dental service use (Wolinsky, 1978: 390). The apparent tendency for the lower social strata to delay in the presentation of symptoms is also well-documented (Koos, 1954: 119; Andersen *et al.*, 1975: 186). Yet, if the relationship between education and utilisation tells us something about the impact of cultural factors, income differences relate more to issues of access and inequality and here there is substantial evidence of income-associated effects on patterns of utilisation (Andersen *et al.,* 1975: 29; Wolinsky, 1978: 390), as there is with more access-related measures such as the dentist: population ratio (Wan and Yates, 1975: 147). Furthermore, once people are actually in the dental system — in other words, once the hurdle of access has been surmounted — neither education nor income exert much influence on the volume of care received (Andersen *et al.,* 1976: 40), a finding that suggests that ease of entry into the dental system is the crucial contingency. This is confirmed, for the USA at least, in the use of medical services; in the study by Taylor *et al.* (1975), the greatest discrepancy between symptoms experienced and practitioner contact occurred for those without access to a regular source of care, independently of race and social-class differences.

The picture is undoubtedly complicated by the fact that few studies of utilisation have traced through the potentially quite different impact of social class on preventive and symptom-related visiting respectively. While preventive activity seems to be more sensitive to cultural factors, one might expect that situational constraints would play a more important part in the process whereby symptoms, once recognised as health needs by the individual, are then translated into effective demand. One of the few attempts to weigh the impact of cultural and situational factors is the work of Kriesberg (1963) and Kriesberg and Treiman (1960). In their reviews of the subject these researchers argue that the supposed social-class differences in cultural attributes, such as attitudes towards dental care and dental utilisation, are not very substantial and that such attitudinal and cultural differences as do exist have a limited, though clearly identifiable, impact on utilisation. When comparing dentistry with other service areas such as medical care, the authors conclude that features of the dental system, especially questions of access to care, have much to do with the persistence of social-class differences since in other areas, such as medicine, social-class differences in utilisation have declined as the system has become more accessible to the disadvantaged.

Conclusion

As they were originally developed in the nineteenth century, the central concepts of epidemiological analysis — age, sex, race and social class — reflect a strikingly different tradition of professional concern to that conventionally espoused by healing practitioners. In contemporary medical practice, the breadth of concern of the practitioner traditionally spreads no further than the individual patient and his ailment, a tradition that is hallowed in a professional mystique regarding the special nature of the relationship between patient and practitioner. Epidemiological method, by its very nature, acknowledges a set of much wider priorities. A concern with the distribution and causes of disease in the community takes the epidemiologist beyond the curative task to consider more preventive forms of health intervention. It also allows for a much franker avowal of the political, institutional and social structural constraints that shape health chances in the community and determine the potential range of strategies of intervention.

The rise of epidemiology and the epidemiological method must be understood within the special historical context of a remarkable series of social and political initiatives in the health field associated with the public health movement of the mid-nineteenth century. The movement was short-lived and failed to establish a philosophy and a set of institutions capable of challenging the orthodoxies of clinical medicine. It is possible to argue that one of the consequences of this failure has been the stunted development of epidemiology itself. The categories of epidemiological analysis live on, of course, but they have lost their 'cutting edge' and have been largely stripped of their earlier social and political significance. While in the nineteenth century epidemiology may have drawn inspiration and meaning from a wider social and political movement in public health, the discipline has since lost its way.

It has been the principal aim of this chapter to attempt to re-establish the links between key epidemiological concepts and a wider framework of social analysis. The most glaring deficiency of the epidemiological approach is its lack of any coherent social theory. In part this is because of the traditional adherence to biological forms of explanation, but it also derives from the traditional eclecticism of epidemiology that has been both its great strength and its weakness. Concepts and terms have been borrowed from other disciplines and applied in an *ad hoc* and untheoretical fashion, with little attempt to integrate them into a broader conceptual framework. The purpose of this chapter, therefore, has been to highlight the non-biological aspects of key epidemiological terms — age and 'social' age, sex and gender, race and ethnicity — and to draw out in a more explicit way the broader understandings of theory and concept in terms of which these notions have to be interpreted. In particular, if there is an overarching framework in which these terms can be located, it is that of social structure. Between them, age, sex, race and

social class form the principal dimensions of a more or less stable
institutional and demographic structure that provides the all-important
social environment for that complex of institutional forms, cultural
practices and patterns of activity that can be called the dental system.

Notes

1. Cited in James and Beal (1974: 79).
2. F.S. McKay began his investigations on fluoride mottling as early as 1908, but the caries inhibitory effects of fluoridation were not fully confirmed till the 1940s (Young and Striffler, 1969: 37-41).
3. Probably the first of its kind was that carried out by Sir John Sinclair on the dental state of 96 old men in 1803 (James and Beal, 1974: 81).
4. Krasner (1978: 25) suggests that the high level of caries attack in the adolescent years can in part be attributed to the rapid physical and emotional changes that are characteristic at this stage of development.
5. Care for these groups tends also to be less remunerative. Feldstein (1977: 83) argues that this is the case for children anyway, and much the same logic would apply for the other groups cited – that is, the time-consuming and demanding nature of the care requirements for such patients.
6. This is confirmed in Koos's (1954: 119) finding that in the city of Regionville in the early 1950s the great majority of children under the age of six, regardless of social background, did not visit the dentist.
7. Sheiham (1977: 443) argues that overtreatment accounts for the tendency for regular attenders to have fewer sound teeth than those who attend on an irregular basis.
8. A widely-held view at this time was that 'to have sound teeth be the mark of a pure Indian and . . . to have carious teeth an indication that there is a strain of white blood in the stock' (cited in Gullett (1971: 5)).
9. On recent British data, the class differentials of the new diseases of affluence have reversed. There are now very few diseases for which the higher socio-economic strata have higher mortality rates (Blaxter, 1976: 113).
10. But, see Kasl and Cobb (1966: 250) where the evidence shows that blacks are actually more likely to take advantage of free health examinations.
11. An example of the operation of gross social and economic disadvantage is Avery's (1976: 19-21) study of migrant and seasonal farmworkers in Florida, 90 per cent of whom were black.
12. For a higher caries prevalence in lower socio-economic strata: Stadt (1967); USPHS (1967a); Koch and Martinsson (1970); Infante and Russell (1974); Holm (1975); Holm *et al.* (1975); Zadik (1978). For studies in which socio-economic status is related to separate DMF components: Richards *et al.* (1965); R. Anderson *et al.* (1971); USPHS (1971); Bagramian and Russell (1973); Antoft *et al.* (1974); USPHS (1974a); Infante and Owen (1975).
13. A study that shows no apparent relationship is Martinsson (1973: 21).
14. See: Kriesberg and Treiman (1962: 42); Kegeles (1963: 97); Rosenstock (1966: 96); Haefner *et al.* (1967: 459); Metz and Richards (1967: 212); Antonovsky and Kats (1970: 372); Jenny *et al.* (1975: 179-84); Nikias *et al.* (1975: 258).

5 CULTURE, LIFE-STYLE AND MODERN SOCIAL PSYCHOLOGY

Unlike the early developments in epidemiology in the public health area, investigators in the dental field have — despite strong biological assumptions inherent in their approach — always taken it for granted that cultural factors and aspects of way of life, such as diet, were important in the etiology and social distribution of oral diseases. By contrast, the theoretical model that the nineteenth-century public-health pioneers of epidemiology developed was one that was much more in keeping with the assumptions of contemporary medical researchers about the workings of acute, infectious diseases. Following the research of Pasteur and the discovery of the microbial carriers of the infectious diseases, it was assumed that the all-important link in the chain of pathology was the infective agent which transmitted a disease from the environment to the host. Hence, the simple epidemiological model of host, agent and environment was developed, and subsequent health strategies organised around this model, involving either the immunisation of the host or the elimination of noxious environmental conditions.

In dentistry, by contrast, it has long been assumed that attributes of the host, like dietary pattern, were important. As early as Aristotle's day, for example, it had been surmised that it was grape-eating that caused caries (Lufkin, 1948: 55), and this kind of thinking has tended to dominate endeavours in the realm of public dental health. Because of the ubiquitous nature of the oral diseases, investigators in the dental field could not make the assumption, as is possible with the infectious diseases, that specific episodes of ill-health follow specific attacks of a disease-carrying agent. Instead, it had to be assumed that the conditions for caries and periodontal disease were more or less constantly present in the population of the industrial societies and that therefore the crucial link in the chain of pathology was not so much the presence of a noxious agent or a disease-carrier, since these were always present, as the susceptibility of the host to pathogens, in its environment, to which it was more or less constantly exposed.

In other words, investigators in the dental field have refined the traditional model of epidemiology in such a way as to adapt it to fit the requirements of chronic, degenerative conditions like caries and periodontal disease. In so-doing they have anticipated developments that have taken place in the broader medical area, as professional thinking and research practice adjust to the requirements of the modern diseases of affluence.[1]

The Politics of Life-Style

Although there has been an appreciation of the importance of diet and personal hygiene practices from the earliest days of dental epidemiology, these factors have tended not to be incorporated in the model in any explicit or fully acknowledged manner. Rather, they have tended to be assumed and taken for granted as essential links in causing oral diseases, and not developed as explanatory terms in their own right. More recently, especially since the 1960s, major changes have taken place in field research so that it is now unusual – rather than the reverse – for an investigator to report a strictly demographic account, in terms of age, sex, race, social class and so on, *without* spelling out the potential impact of attitudes and behaviour patterns.

There are two major reasons for this change. Firstly, it was evident to investigators that the standard demographic account was yielding rapidly diminishing returns in both theoretical understanding and the potential for policy intervention. The demographic tradition pointed to social-structural factors that were relatively stable and unchanging, and certainly unresponsive to initiatives for change of any ordinary political dimensions (Becker, 1974: 409). It therefore seemed reasonable to develop those areas of research where there was at least some prospect for change in the short term, and this seems to have been the primary motivation of social psychologists and some sociologists working on the impact of attitudes and health beliefs on personal care and service utilisation.

A second major reason for these shifts in theoretical emphasis relates to wider social and political changes and the consequences of these changes for the position of the dental profession in the advanced industrial societies. In fact, the issue is of much wider relevance, affecting not only the interests of dentistry, but also those of medicine and the allied health professions and probably the whole range of human service occupations as well. The critical situation in the wider health field arises from a quite simple combination of circumstances. On the one hand there has been an extremely rapid increase in the commitment of resources to health care, in most countries doubling over the last decade, with increases in real terms of 30-100 per cent (Michel, 1974:

12). These increases have not been matched by any corresponding improvement in life expectancy or health chances (McKinlay and
McKinlay, 1977), and have taken place at a time when it is becoming
increasingly apparent that the rules of orthodox economic theory do
not necessarily hold unchallenged in the health area.[2]

On the other hand, there has arisen a climate of public expectation
and concern about: improved access to care; the effectiveness of medical
procedures; and rationality and economy in the deployment of health
resources. Nor are such concerns restricted to an intellectual *avant garde*
outside the profession. An indication that such ideas have 'arrived' in
professional circles was given by the wide publicity accorded an address
by Dr Mahler (the director of WHO), since published in the *Lancet*
(Mahler, 1978). He accused the medical establishment of manipulating
developments in medical care in a direction that was contrary to the
broader public interest. In particular, he castigated the profession's
'mystification' of health issues and its failure to cultivate public understanding.

It is in such circumstances — of rising costs, diminishing returns to investment in health, growing public expectation and political pressure —
that a new consensus has emerged in the profession, the object of which
has been to reconcile these external pressures with the traditional health
concerns of medical practitioners. The response in both the USA
(Knowles, 1977) and in the UK (DHSS, 1976) has been to stress the
responsibility of individuals for their own health. Similar events have
occurred in dentistry. In recent years both the British and American
dental associations have sponsored quite major reports on the problematic attitudes and motivations of the poor and the disadvantaged
(Scarrott, 1969; Bureau of Economic Research and Statistics, 1958),
thus hoping to swing the terms of research away from sensitive issues in
the organisation and delivery of care.[3]

Of course, much research in the life-style tradition reflects the influence of academic social psychology, but it also reflects a more or less
realistic appraisal of the options for intervention. Such is the limited
potential for change in the dental system that researchers have naturally
considered strategies that by-pass the need for any major restructuring
of the established delivery system. An indication of the lengths to which
researchers have gone in this line of research is the work of Reiss *et al.*
(1976) on different methods of encouraging low-income parents to seek
dental care for their children. Rather than considering ways in which the
system might be changed in order to achieve higher levels of utilisation
among the poor, attention has instead been directed at the poor them-

selves, as if some aspect of personality or value system were at fault. Ironically, in the case of this study the most effective inducement to seeking dental care was monetary; those parents with the inducement of a five-dollar reward were much more likely to contact the dentist than those prompted by a phone call and a home visit.

On the one hand, then, is the tradition of social research in which investigators have made a more or less realistic assessment of the prospects for change and, given the dominant influence in the USA of modern social psychology, have come to concentrate their attentions on the modification of key beliefs and attitudes. On the other hand, and complementary to this tradition, are those trends in research and debate encouraged by considerations of professional interest. Against a background of rising public expectations and growing political pressure, spokesmen of organised dentistry have been concerned to foster public debate and academic research that concentrates on issues of attitude and education, rather than on questions of manpower structure, the organisation and delivery of care, alternative payment systems and the accessibility of services. Between them, modern social psychology and professional interests have together gone far to encourage an emphasis on attitudes and life-styles that dominates much contemporary thinking in oral health care.

The Effects of Diet

It is probably no exaggeration to say that, because its prevalence in affluent, urban populations has long been linked to aspects of life-style, and to diet in particular, caries was one of the first acknowledged modern 'diseases of civilisation'. While there is much evidence of a circumstantial nature linking life-style to dental health, there are also carefully controlled studies that provide more convincing proof of the impact of modern diet on the development of caries. The circumstantial evidence is plentiful, but much of it relies on the rather questionable logic of assuming that, because two factors can empirically be shown to vary together over time and place, they are therefore linked in a relationship of cause and effect.[4] There is plenty of evidence of this type associating the advent of modern diet — and modern institutions generally — to changes in oral health; some of these have been in the virtual form of 'natural experiments', e.g. the study of the Scottish island of Lewis (Burman, 1964; Hargreaves, 1972), and a similar one carried out on the population of the island of Tristan da Cunha

(P. Holloway *et al.,* 1963).

The very special circumstances of reduced sugar intake in wartime Europe provided research conditions that are even closer to those of the laboratory experiment since, unlike the two island studies, the effects of dietary changes can be isolated from the possible impact of other aspects of modern life. In all of the European countries affected by the Second World War, the consumption of sugar fell quite dramatically for a period, and then returned to its former level. Such unusually good experimental conditions would seem to provide an ideal opportunity to establish the link between sugar and caries. Even under these favourable conditions, however, the interpretation of the data has been challenged. While Toverud(1957) and Marthaler (1967) claim to show that the caries incidence fell as a result of wartime restrictions on diet, Wandelt (1969) provides data showing that, as in the rest of Europe, dental caries fell in Berlin during the War, but that this decrease was not associated with any corresponding change in the levels of sugar consumption. Jackson (1974) and Glass *et al.* (1973) are other researchers who, after various statistical manipulations of the data, claim that caries did not fall over the wartime period, or, at least, not in any way or to any extent that can be linked to the drop in sugar consumption. Of all the studies on the sugar-caries link, only the classic Vipeholm research (Gustafsson *et al.,* 1954) has managed, outside laboratory conditions, to isolate and measure the precise cariogenic effects of various sucrose elements in the diet.

More recently there have been a number of field studies that have investigated the relationship between diet and caries, but results so far have been rather inconclusive. Recent American research using social-survey techniques has failed to show any relationship between the consumption of snacks and caries levels (Bagramian and Russell, 1973; Bagramian *et al.,* 1974; Clancey *et al.,* 1977; 1978). A basic methodological flaw in most of these studies is their dependence on the analysis of data collected at only one point in time. Since caries is cumulative, and patterns of snacking can change over time, information collected at a single timepoint can clearly be misleading. But even a longitudinal study carried out by Glass and Fleish (1974) over a period of two years failed to establish any association between the consumption of breakfast cereals and caries increase. A number of South African studies also report inconsistent results (Retief *et al.,* 1975; Richardson *et al.,* 1978a; 1978b).

To be set alongside these negative results, however, there are at least as many other diet inventory studies that report statistical associations, none of them very striking, between consumption patterns – eating and drinking potentially cariogenic items – and caries (Mansbridge, 1960;

Koch and Martinsson, 1971; Samuelson *et al.,* 1971; Duany *et al.,* 1972; Hankin *et al.,* 1973; Martinsson, 1973; Holm *et al.,* 1975; Ringelberg and Tonascia, 1976). The mechanism of such cariogenic effects may be quite subtle. An example, Anaise's (1978) study of workers in the Israeli sweet industry shows evidence of higher DMF levels and suggests that this greater risk can be traced both to the direct consumption of sweets and also to the pollution of the work atmosphere by carbohydrates.

Anaise's work is just one of a number of recent studies that seem to confirm the sugar-caries link, in the light of which one is tempted to enquire as to why it is that so many other studies appear to point to the opposite conclusion. Part of the reason for this apparent discrepancy may well be methodological. None of these studies has been able to replicate the carefully controlled experimental conditions that Gustafsson *et al.* (1954) were able to create in their field research at Vipeholm, and the alternative — laboratory studies using animals or artificial devices — provides data that cannot necessarily be generalised to human dietary patterns in the real world (Allman, 1971).

Another factor that may account for the inconsistent results on caries and sugar is the possibility that modern diets are already so high in sugar content that the relationship between sugar intake and caries becomes obscured above a certain threshold level of sucrose in the diet (King, 1978: 47). Another possibility, as Bibby (1975) argues, is that the form and manner in which cariogenic items are consumed is more important than any simple measure of the level of sugar content. Therefore, studies that use a simple summary measure of snack consumption, for example, may well be failing to obtain a true assessment of their cariogenic potential.

Culture and Preventive Health Behaviour

The relationship between diet and caries provides a clear example of the importance of the cultural perspective in epidemiological analysis. The case of periodontal disease, however, introduces questions of a rather different order since diet, which provides a firm link with culture in the case of caries, is of little importance here (Russell, 1963: 242; Schonfeld, 1963: 931). This is not to say that behavioural factors exert no influence on the periodontal condition. They do. But the impact of culture and life-style on periodontal disease is rather different from the effect of such factors in the case of caries. Diet is culturally sanctioned, of course, and, as such, its impact on the behaviour of the individual is something that occurs at a more or less subliminal or subconscious level. Diet is merely one attribute in a broader cultural pattern. Like many other aspects of the way of life of whole societies or communities it is taken for granted. While it may be regarded as a risk behaviour by the observer, it is certainly not consciously viewed as such by the individual – at least under normal circumstances. It is just part of an accepted pattern of life. The potential for conscious, preventive health activity is therefore rather limited. The periodontal condition, however, seems to be affected by a range of more consciously initiated activities that have no counterpart in the control of caries.

Certainly, there is evidence from a number of controlled school-studies that professional cleaning and oral hygiene programmes produce marked reductions in caries activity (Agerback *et al.,* 1977; Helöe and König, 1978), a result that argues for the importance of conscious, preventive action in the case of tooth decay. In many instances, however, there remains the considerable methodological difficulty of separating out, on the one hand, the effects of oral hygiene instruction and professional cleaning, from the impact of fluoride applications of various kinds on the other (Marthaler, 1972a; 1972b; Lindhe *et al.,* 1975; Bennie *et al.,* 1976; Hamp *et al.,* 1978). In one study that managed to isolate the effects of the different components of the intervention programme – and, in particular, was able to remove the effect of fluoride applications – caries activity was found to *increase* with normal plaque control activities in the absence of topical fluoride application (Axelsson *et al.,* 1976: 238). But even if we accept those school studies that appear to highlight the success of oral hygiene in controlling caries, it has then to be acknowledged that in most cases the measured improvements in health status did not long outlast the termination of the programme (Lindhe and Koch, 1967; Berenie *et al.,* 1976; Horowitz *et al.,* 1977).

Therefore, while there is certainly evidence that personal care activities can make some impact on caries, the conditions under which these research results have been obtained make them of doubtful application in the field. [5] In this respect periodontal disease is in a different category. The impact of cultural factors is limited to a range of consciously initiated personal activities, while in the case of caries broader life-style attributes are important. This suggests a significant difference in approach to the analysis of social behaviour in this area; it also has important implications for the contrasting policy strategies entailed by these two conditions.

Unlike caries, then, the periodontal condition is affected by behaviour that is more consciously initiated and motivated, and it is in this area that the bulk of the work on life-style has been carried out. Perhaps the clearest example of this philosophy at work is in health education since it is here, more than in the case of diet, that particular patterns of preventive activity can be encouraged. Health education appears to offer the opportunity to impart information and attitudes about aspects of behaviour affecting the individual's health. As long as one can make the assumption that certain health-related aspects of behaviour can be treated as more or less consciously and rationally initiated, then imparting information about health activities — such as personal oral hygiene and preventive dental visiting — appears to be a valid strategy. An example of a dental health education package recently marketed in the USA is the so-called 'Toothkeeper' programme, a programme that has been evaluated in a number of school intervention studies (Graves *et al.,* 1975; Smith *et al.,* 1975; Stamm *et al.,* 1975). In none of these studies has the programme been demonstrated to have any significant effect, thus largely confirming the pessimistic conclusion reached by Frazier (1978) in a wide-ranging review of the dental health education literature. Furthermore, even where such programmes do appear to make some impact, there is very often a rapid fall-off in information retention after the end of the programme (Addy and Edmunds, 1977: 193), though this effect may vary by age (Rayner and Cohen, 1977: 65).

In practice it is very difficult — if not artificial — to separate items of behaviour (e.g. health information and preventive activity), that are consciously directed towards health maintenance and can to some extent be isolated, *from* other activities less consciously initiated and more closely interwoven into a broader cultural pattern. Furthermore, this difficulty in separating these two different forms of behaviour may go some way to explaining why health education programmes have had such limited success. A number of studies have shown, for example, that the health knowledge and practices of lower socio-economic strata compare unfavourably with those of the middle class (Pratt, 1971: 289; Dennison, 1972: 819). Is it therefore the policy implication, that these aspects of lower-class life can, and should, be isolated from their broader cultural context and changed by disseminating the correct information and attitudes?

The evidence, though largely impressionistic, is that such items are rather difficult to alter individually, and in isolation, if only because they are usually quite closely interwoven with wider cultural patterns. To a greater or lesser extent the sub-cultures of different social strata are relatively consistent within themselves and represent more or less successful adaptations to different social and economic conditions. It is therefore difficult to imagine being able to identify certain items in a given sub-culture, grouping them together as 'health activities' and then successfully treating them in isolation from their cultural context. The range of everyday activities that have important implications for personal health is rather striking. The research of Breslow and Belloc has shown, for example, that taking just seven basic health practices one can account for quite a significant amount of variation in illness and mortality in any given population (Belloc and Breslow, 1972; Breslow, 1972; Belloc, 1973). Nor are these practices unusual patterns of behaviour that might mark them out from any other everyday activity; they include eight hours sleep, regular meals, some physical activity, and limited smoking and drinking, none of which need appear to be overtly and strongly related to health promotion.

It is unlikely that anything more than a handful of people consciously carry out such activities for reasons of health alone. As Baric (1969) points out, in contrast to the role of sick person or patient, which is firmly defined and has a well-established pattern of social expectation associated with it, the idea that an individual might be 'at risk' from certain health hazards is one that receives very little cultural support. The fact that certain activities are hazardous to health is not something that is reinforced consistently by health authorities, or by the individual's environment, nor can it be based on the perception of any concrete symptoms or professional activities. Nor does it entail any acknowledged rights and duties towards others. Instead, health hazards — and their converse, preventive health activities — are items of behaviour that are not often isolated and consciously identified as being relevant to the tasks of health maintenance and health promotion.

Many activities with important repercussions for personal health, then, may not be culturally acknowledged or identified as such. But the fact that many such actions are carried out and embedded within a wider cultural context that does not necessarily formally acknowledge their relevance to health does not mean that they will not, or cannot, change in piecemeal fashion. After all, the novel health behaviour of today can become the firmly established cultural pattern of tomorrow, as in the case of toothbrushing which is now a virtually universal practice (Cohen *et al.,* 1967: 230), firmly embedded in daily grooming routines.

In fact, it is a defensible proposition that our health education efforts of the past have been rather too successful, not the reverse, since much of the misinformation that the public today holds about dental health and dental care can be traced directly to notions that were once prevalent in the profession and which we now know to be false. Many popular notions about dental care can be traced back to ideas that were at one time current in professional circles and that were more or less successfully disseminated to the public, which suggests that health-related behaviour can and does change as a result of health information becoming more widely available.[6] Similarly, there is little doubt that risk behaviours that seem to be firmly embedded in wider patterns of behaviour can in fact be tackled in a piecemeal fashion, and in the short-term also, by legislative action and various economic rewards and punishments.[7]

It is such on examples of successful legislative initiatives, and on the evidence of the impact of earlier professional ideas on popular dental beliefs and practices, that investigators have based the assumption that many practices wittingly or unwittingly related to health can be changed without wholesale re-fashioning of a broader cultural context. It is this belief that inspires much of the work on attitudes and life-styles in contemporary health services research. In this respect the case of dentistry is rather unique since, more than many other areas, the oral condition is clearly affected by a range of activities, some of them — such as toothbrushing and visiting the dentist — culturally acknowledged as health practices, others — such as diet — less formally so, but all recognised by professionals at least for their importance to health. In this respect, personal dental care, and its underlying philosophy of prevention, has provided something of a model for researchers in the field.

The Health Beliefs Model

Although it has not in any way been formally incorporated into social research in dentistry, Baric's (1969) concept of the 'at risk' role shares much common ground with the preventive philosophy that underlies personal dental care and also provides a framework for its analysis. Central to Baric's notion of the 'at risk' role is the idea that the host — in the orthodox epidemiological triad of host, agent and environment — is no longer to be viewed as an innocent victim of his or her environment, as is the natural assumption with the traditional infectious diseases, but instead is to be regarded as actively involved in the disease process itself, to the extent of actually affecting its onset and the course of its development. In other words, in this conception, disease is no longer to be seen as an 'accident' of exposure to a hazardous environment, but as a maladjustment to an environment that is more or less constantly exposing the individual to various health risks. Suchman (1970:

105-6) and Richards (1975: 144), from this reconstructed epidemiological model, see the environment as something that is almost a constant source of hazard, i.e. ill-health is not an accident but a statistical certainty, unless the individual can take the necessary precautions. Hence, in this view, failures of perception, information or motivation account for much of the impact of the modern diseases of affluence.

It is this subtle shift in the focus of the epidemiological framework that lies at the base of much of the research on life-styles in health, especially the work in the tradition of what has come to be called the Health Beliefs Model (HBM). At the centre of the model is the assumption that much individual behaviour in the health field can be understood in terms of the costs and benefits that individuals face in considering various courses of action that are open to them. These costs and benefits are, of course, subjective and are weighed in the light of various beliefs that individuals may have about their health and how to maintain it. Therefore, if a person is concerned about his susceptibility to a particular condition, a condition which he views as a potentially serious threat to his health, and if he can see the possible benefits accruing from appropriate health action, then there will be a very high probability of that action being taken. It is often further assumed that this action requires some identifiable cue or 'trigger' for health beliefs to be translated into effective behaviour.

Essentially, this is a model of individual decision-making and, as such, has a certain generality, i.e. it can be applied across a whole range of preventive activities, including screening and visiting for health checks. In principle it can be extended to any area where the individual has to weight the consequences of different courses of action, including those frequent occasions when the individual has to consider whether or not to seek aid for symptoms. In this respect the model applies equally in the field of dentistry as it does in medicine since, despite the prevailing ethos of prevention, symptomatic visiting is almost as important a pattern of utilisation in dentistry as it is in the case of medical care.[8] Despite this potential generality of the model, however, it still remains true that most work carried out in the HBM tradition has concerned areas of preventive action rather than symptom-related behaviour.

A number of studies have now been carried out within the HBM framework, in the main with rather mixed success. In one of the earlier reviews of the work carried out in this area, Rosenstock (1966) concluded from research on the use of preventive and detection services that, while the findings on the role of health beliefs were largely in the direction predicted by the model, and were more or less consistent across

different types of service, including preventive dental care, the evidence
for the model was not entirely persuasive because it was so weakly, if
also consistently, supported. At about the same time a national survey
of health beliefs in the USA — reported by Haefner *et al.* (1967) —
collected a far more comprehensive and representative set of information
on four preventive health actions, including toothbrushing and preventive dental visiting. The survey established that there was a considerable
degree of consistency of behaviour across different types of health
action, with those who were preventively inclined in one area tending
also to report one or more of the other preventive activities. There was
also some consistency over time since a preventive action, once taken,
was likely to be repeated at some future date.

Another study shortly after the national survey, reported by Tash *et
al.* (1969), produced mixed results. Contrary to the predictions of the
model it found that those who felt less susceptible to dental problems
were in fact more, not less, likely to use the dentist preventively,
possibly because those receiving more care felt a greater confidence
about the state of their dental health. The perceived seriousness of
dental problems, and a belief in the efficacy of dental visiting, both contributed to a higher rate of preventive visiting, as predicted by the
model, though in neither case was the relationship very strong. Cost and
fear of pain were seen as barriers to visiting. Becker *et al.* (1972; 1977a),
in placing health beliefs within a framework of patient compliance with
medical regimens, have given the HBM a slightly different emphasis. Although the interest is still in health actions with a major preventive
emphasis — child health; diet — the significance of health beliefs in their
work is in affecting compliance with specific regimens, rather than in the
prediction of the use of preventive services. Others have looked at the
impact of health beliefs on the non-preventive use of medical services
(Kirscht *et al.,* 1976; Leavitt, 1979). These studies show that, after illness symptoms have been taken into account, and in circumstances
where the normal barriers of cost and access have been substantially
reduced, the effect of health beliefs in predicting levels of utilisation
comes through very clearly.

What conclusions can we draw from the research that has been carried
out in the HBM tradition, especially in the context of dental care? We
are now in a better position to assess the contribution of health beliefs
research since in recent years the principle researchers involved in work
in the HBM tradition have produced a number of articles reviewing the
effect of beliefs on dental behaviour. Haefner (1974) argues that the
research to date does not provide definitive evidence that health beliefs

influence preventive dental behaviour, since most studies tend to provide a mixture of both negative and positive results. Kegeles (1974a), writing at the same time, attempts to identify those areas where he thinks that health beliefs do have some predictive usefulness. His conclusion is that in certain combinations – perceptions of susceptibility and severity of a condition, and the belief in the efficacy and benefit of action – health beliefs make a significant impact on regular dental utilisation and tooth-brushing; taken individually, these factors have almost no effect on preventive dental behaviour.

Elsewhere Kegeles (1974b; 1975) considers in more detail the potential impact on preventive health actions of beliefs about susceptibility to dental problems. In the case of people's beliefs about their possible susceptibility to caries, there appears to be no relationship between dental visiting or brushing and the prevention of tooth decay, though it is unlikely that people brush their teeth without some trust in its effectiveness. Concern about 'serious dental problems', on the other hand, does seem to be associated with periodic, preventive visiting, a finding that provides at least some confirmation of the importance of perceptions of susceptibility to health problems. This is further supported by Becker *et al.* (1977b) who argue that beliefs about susceptibility to dental problems provide the strongest evidence for the model. In a review of the literature, Becker and Maiman (1975) conclude in a generally more optimistic vein than Kegeles. They are able to find much more support for the influence of health beliefs, especially where a number of such beliefs are associated together and especially where compliance with health recommendations on dental care are considered.

The Limitations of the Model

No matter how optimistic a view we take on the research to date, the evidence for the HBM is, at best, mildly favourable, but in general rather inconclusive. Questions of methodology apart, one possible conclusion that we may be able to draw from these results is that the rationalistic assumptions of the model are at fault. It is quite possible that people do not in fact approach health behaviour in the rationalistic, decision-making manner portrayed in the HBM, at least in the absence of major sanctions, or cues to action (such as physical coercion or substantial economic or psychological rewards and punishments). After all, we know enough about the behaviour of smokers to recognise that individuals can reconcile and compartmentalise quite inconsistent information;

smokers know about the horrors of lung cancer and its relationship to smoking, but they are able to balance this information against other needs and beliefs that outweigh the immediate concern with health (Kirscht, 1974: 467). Therefore, if the health beliefs framework applies at all, it may well apply only in those areas of behaviour where very specific motivations and beliefs address quite specific forms of activity; in such areas of behaviour it is probably also easier to identify, detach and then modify beliefs sufficiently to change the associated activities. Where actions satisfy a variety of needs and motivations it is not possible to isolate and change beliefs and actions in this way, and the underlying notion of rational decision-making that underlies the health beliefs methodology is inadequate.

Even where it is possible to specify a health action in such a way that we can associate clearly identifiable beliefs and motivations with it, there still remains the question as to whether such beliefs precede and moti-vate health behaviour, or whether the reverse is the case. Although it has come as a natural assumption for many researchers in the health beliefs area that beliefs and attitudes precede and motivate action, there is evid-ence that the converse is also true. For example, in their study of the preventive utilisation of dentists' services among teenagers, Kriesberg and Treiman (1962) found that the strong relationship between family socio-economic status and preventive visiting could not be accounted for by the general dental orientations, attitudes and beliefs of the teenagers themselves. This relationship between beliefs and utilisation held for the adults in the study and, even more strongly, for the relationship between adult beliefs and teenage patterns of visiting.

Assuming that the generation of teenagers studied by Kriesberg and Treiman are going to continue the cycle of socio-economic advantage and disadvantage by emulating their parents in much the same way as previous generations, then what this information suggests is that, given the correct social circumstances, patterns of behaviour – in this case, preventive visiting – can become well-established in advance of the usual set of supporting beliefs and attitudes. This result is obtained not only through the direct influence of parents on the dental visiting patterns of their children, but also through the parental choice of dentist since, according to Kriesberg and Treiman, those teenagers (and adults) with dentists who were preventively inclined in their dental practice tended also to use the dentist in a preventive manner.

This last point introduces a further dimension into any evaluation of the HBM framework, since the role of the dentist, and the importance of the patient-practitioner relationship, are not easily accommodated because they suggest that a person's use of dental services may be guided by their relationship with the dental system just as much as by their beliefs and attitudes. In fact, Kasl and Cobb (1966) go so far as to argue that much utilisation is better viewed as a more or less stable pattern of behaviour or a habit, rather than a series of discrete events as it is so apt to be seen within the HBM framework. In other words, it should be viewed as the use and re-use of an established patient-practitioner relationship, rather than a search for aid embarked upon *de novo* on each occasion. The introduction of 'the dental system' into the model allows us to consider another possibility that is otherwise rather implausible within the health beliefs framework; that is, that individuals may hold the appropriate or favourable dental attitudes, but be unable or unwilling for one reason or another to translate such beliefs into effective action. Obviously there is a great range of potential barriers, not all of which may be clearly acknowledged or articulated by the dental consumer. But it is at least plausible that such barriers may account for some of the rather weak and inconsistent findings in HBM research. And it is quite possible that the barriers we are thinking of are rather few in number. Freidson and Feldman (1958: 334-5), for example, attribute this gap between knowledge and practice to economic and time costs and fear of pain.

As these last examples suggest, the other major defect of the health beliefs approach is its radically social-psychological term of reference. The fact that knowledge does not necessarily translate into the appropriate action may be related to a host of barriers that exist outside the individual; in dentistry these may be problems of access and cost, as well as fear of pain. The expectation in HBM research is that such obstacles and barriers can be clearly articulated by people and related to their health actions. But this may not always be the case. Partly this is a question of faulty methodology and unrealistic expectations as to what can be extracted from survey research. But partly it may also be a matter of what standards and expectations people bring to dental care. If the goal — adequate dental care — is something for which a person cannot or does not realistically aspire, then potential barriers may not be viewed as obstacles to care.

This concept of reference groups external to a person, setting standards of aspiration for them and providing sounding boards for them to evaluate their health and the standard of care received, is something that is difficult to insert in the HBM framework (Jaccard, 1975: 165). Furthermore, just as reference groups set standards — in the light of tradition and the realities of access — so such groups play an important part in enforcing individual conformity to these standards. So, even where we know that certain group standards or norms exist — standards that may exert an effect quite independently of the individual's health beliefs — we still cannot judge their potential impact on the individual's behaviour without knowing something further about the cohesiveness of the group and its ability to enforce conformity with its standards, since the greater the cohesion of the group, the greater the likelihood that individuals will respond to medical problems in a way that is consistent with the health values of their group (Geertsen *et al.,* 1975: 233). Again, this will be a factor that may operate quite independently of the individual's expressed health beliefs as reported in a survey interview.

A particularly concrete manifestation of this kind of group pressure is the influence that social networks may have on individual behaviour, including preventive health activity. In one recent study (Langlie, 1977: 254) the combined effects of health beliefs and social-structural factors, including social networks, accounted for 40 per cent of the reported variation in patterns of preventive health behaviour. In another study, that assessed the impact of demographic and social-psychological factors on dental utilisation, the effects of health beliefs and knowledge were limited compared to the impact of access and broader sub-cultural factors (Wan and Yates, 1975: 146-7), which again underlines the importance of community context in encouraging particular kinds of behaviour quite independently of individual attitudes and beliefs.

The Culture of Dentistry

Attitudes and behaviour, therefore, cannot be isolated from their cultural context without doing violence to the manifold complexity and interrelatedness of everyday life. Just as a risk behaviour such as smoking is embedded within a wider life-style, so various health practices must be understood within a rich and varied historical and social context. The advent of high quality restorative and preventive dentistry has been relatively recent and, furthermore, as it has become available it has been concentrated among social groups that are socially and economically advantaged in a number of ways, quite apart from their access to dental services.[9] Therefore, for a disadvantaged population with a folk memory of emergency dental treatment received under trying conditions and with limited local access, the development of preventive orientations to dental care may make little sense. Furthermore, where such values *do* emerge, the chances of their being translated into effective action are limited.

In other words, cultural attributes – like attitudes to dental health and dental care – have to be viewed as aspects of a broader framework of shared understandings about accepted forms of behaviour in many different areas of life. A chronic, non-fatal and, in the view of many, inevitable condition like caries or periodontal disease may not merit the special attention that more serious health problems like cancer and heart disease receive. Therefore, while there *are* clearly understandings specific to dentistry – a lay culture of dentistry perhaps – such understandings may be relatively latent and, in any case, have to be interpreted within the wider context of group life and the existence of other culturally sanctioned beliefs and practices.

The life-style concept and the HBM are both developments that have retarded, rather than advanced, our understanding of the lay culture of dentistry. Life-style because, in its popular interpretation at least, it reduces values, beliefs and activities to the level of more or less voluntarily chosen attributes of living. The implication of the life-style approach is that, just as a person may choose to exhibit a certain manner and style of living – especially in the realm of consumer goods – so, by analogy, they may also choose to carry out certain preventive health activities, adding them to their repertoire of behaviour. If it is then possible, the reasoning continues, to trace the sources of motivation for such choices, then, by judicious intervention with health education campaigns, etc. it is possible to encourage healthier ways of living. Such seems to be the logic of the life-style approach to health-related activities.

The HBM also follows a similarly individualistic approach to health-related behaviour. While it does not have the connotations of a personally selected, or at least accepted, range of beliefs and practices, it does suggest that everything that needs to be known about the individual's health-related activities can be understood by taking a social-psychological inventory of attitudes and behaviour. Given such an inventory, one can then plan forms of intervention that foster the right set of beliefs and practices. In particular, if only certain strategic health beliefs can be modified in the right direction, then the appropriate health actions will follow.

Of course, there *are* elements of unconstrained choice in people's health actions. Moreover, there must obviously be much that can be understood about the pattern of such activities by reference merely to certain pertinent beliefs about health hazards, such as susceptibility, seriousness and appropriate action. But, at the same time, people's choices, beliefs and activities have to be viewed within a wider cultural context. It is this broader pattern of accepted values, attitudes and practices that sets the framework within which individuals think and act. Furthermore, it is these values and practices with a more general and abstract point of reference that provide the cultural background for the development of forms of belief and behaviour that are specific to health.

Therefore, central to the concept of culture is the interrelatedness of different spheres of social action. At the core of a culture of dentistry may be beliefs and practices that are very specific to dental care and dental health, but these overlap with broader health concerns and values. These in turn articulate with yet wider cultural forms. There is thus a limit to the extent to which specific items of life-style and belief can be modified without related changes in other areas of life. Furthermore, because these items represent a cultural adaptation to aspects of an encompassing social and economic environment, there are environmental constraints on change as well. This environment represents a social reality against which cultural attributes are tested, adapted and developed. If values, beliefs and practices are too much at variance with the realities of health care — for example, if there are difficulties in obtaining high quality dental care at a reasonable price — then they will be discarded.[10] It is by this emphasis on the interrelatedness of different aspects of group life that the concept of culture does so much to modify the claims made for modern social psychology in social science research in dentistry.

Notes

1. Richards (1975: 143-4) argues that the transition from the bacteriological era of the nineteenth century to the contemporary diseases of civilisation has had a profound impact on our conceptual framework.

2. Supply seems to create demand; output is difficult to assess; there does not seem to be any 'natural equilibrium' between supply and demand; consumers are not knowledgeable about the product they are purchasing; and in many instances 'money is no object' where questions of life and death are concerned (Michel, 1974: 11). For evidence on the limited returns to medical intervention, see: McKeown (1976: 7-9); McKinlay and McKinlay (1977: 425).

3. Such is the 'victim-blaming' tenor of much research that one observer has been moved to comment that the dictum of many investigators must be 'to the victim belong all the flaws' (Galanter, 1977: 1025).

4. For example, Hardwick (1960: 16-17).

5. One study in which toothbrushing seemed to reduce the increase in caries is Leske *et al.* (1976).

6. The great majority of people, for example, believe that toothbrushing 'fights tooth decay', a sentiment that has been assiduously cultivated by the advertising

industry and that at one time accurately reflected the state of professional opinion on the matter, but a statement that nevertheless we now know to be incorrect (Cohen *et al.,* 1967: 234; O'Shea and Gray, 1968: 409). Also, although people know of periodontal disease, they have little knowledge that associates it with poor oral hygiene, a state of ignorance that follows closely upon years of uncertainty on the question even in well-informed professional circles (Linn, 1965: 41).

7. One example cited by Terris (1967: 2088) is the reduction in cirrhosis of the liver in the UK, in marked contrast to the situation in the USA, a change which he attributes to the policy of high alcohol prices that has been followed in Britain but not in America.

8. According to the WHO cross-national study of medical care carried out in a number of areas across seven countries, 24 per cent of dental visits were for check-ups, compared to 19 per cent of visits to medical practitioners (Kohn and White, 1976).

9. In the USA three-quarters of all dental visits are accounted for by 18 per cent of the population and three-quarters of all dental expenditure is attributable to just 10 per cent (Schoen, 1978: 186-7).

10. The idea that circumstances of economic and social disadvantage will shape and form associated values, attitudes and aspirations is central to the concept of the 'culture of poverty' (Rodman, 1977: 867). This concept has lost favour with some because of the way in which it has been used to turn the tables on the poor – 'blaming the victim' – in characterising the socially and economically disadvantaged as deficient in certain middle-class attributes (McKinlay, 1972). The value of the concept lies in the clear policy implication that any attempt to change attitudes and values without also altering broader social and economic barriers and constraints is bound to fail.

THE PROFESSIONAL CULTURE OF DENTISTRY

One thing that emerges clearly from any review of the literature on what people think and do about oral health and oral care is the great variability in beliefs and practices that exists among different social groups. These variations are probably no greater than they are in other areas of life such as politics, education, religion, health and domestic life-style, but it is striking nevertheless to find the sort of diversity that characterises, for example, the way in which different ethnic groups and social-class strata use dental services. Although there is this social diversity in dentistry, as there is in any other area of health, it is possible nevertheless to identify certain common tendencies, certain shared dental beliefs and practices that one would be justified in calling a 'lay culture of dentistry'. Furthermore, insofar as we can talk of such a folk culture, it is clear that it contains many elements of belief and practice that are at some variance with professional opinion, especially in the case of those social strata that do not have ready access to, and extensive informal contact with, the professional upper middle class.

In some respects it is remarkable the extent to which certain items of professional teaching are so widely disseminated in the population. Toothbrushing, for example, is now almost universally practised in the advanced industrial societies, a testimony perhaps to growing health consciousness, but more likely a social trend that has been greatly aided by the efforts of commercial interests. A major stimulus was probably the advent of commercial dentifrices, or toothpastes, since it was only then that oral cleanliness became palatable and pleasant,[1] as well as something that contributed to oral health. The demands of aesthetic appeal have probably also been important in contributing to the wide acceptance of toothbrushing.

Paradoxically, if studies in the USA are any guide, when asked for possible health reasons for brushing their teeth, people tended to give answers that were not supported by current professional opinion on the question. While the accepted view in dentistry is that toothbrushing may have some effect in preventing periodontal disease, as may regular visits to the dentist, there is very limited evidence that either of these practices contributes to the control of caries. Yet it is the prevention of tooth decay that, according to interview surveys on the subject, motivates the great majority of people to brush their teeth (Cohen *et al.*,

1967: 230-4; O'Shea and Gray, 1968: 409).

In practice, of course, it may not matter that people are carrying out health activities for what might be regarded as the 'wrong' reasons. The effect is going to be the same regardless of motivation or intent. But ironically, what we now see as the popular mythology of today was in fact the firmly held professional belief of yesterday. These very same views on the effectiveness of toothbrushing that we now know to be incorrect were at one time the conventional wisdom of dental practice. What appears to be happening in this instance, as in other areas of health, is that professional opinions and beliefs take some time to become fully diffused in the population. With advances in research and with shifts in intellectual fashion, professional opinion changes, and so the whole cycle of diffusion and dissemination begins again. Meanwhile, of course, there is a considerable 'culture lag' between popular beliefs and the state of opinion in the profession itself.

Further evidence of 'culture lag' in the dissemination of health information is provided in recent survey data from Finland. In two major surveys Markkula *et al.* (1977) found that those most likely to believe that oral hygiene makes the greatest contribution to the prevention and control of caries were the young, the well-educated and urban dwellers, precisely those groups that one would expect to be among the best-informed. In contrast, those who felt that the consumption of sugar had most to do with caries and its prevention were the old, the less-educated and those living in rural areas, just those groups that one would expect to be less well-informed on the subject. What at first appears to be a rather paradoxical finding may well be explicable in terms of the same 'culture lag' phenomenon. While those from an earlier generation of dental practice still believe in the simple verities of diet, those exposed to a more recent health message profess a more sophisticated understanding of caries etiology and prevention that gives a prominent place to personal care and preventive activity.

There is similar evidence of an information lag in the case of periodontal disease. Although a high percentage of people can recognise the principal symptoms of gum problems (Cohen *et al.*, 1967: 242; Ainamo, 1972: 615; Markkula *et al.*, 1977: 112), few are able to apply this to the extent of actually being able to assess correctly their own periodontal condition (Vogan, 1970: 482; Murtomaa and Ainamo, 1977: 197). In fact, there is some evidence that for certain social groups 'bleeding gums' may be accepted as a normal condition of the mouth. In Vogan's study of 300 office and factory workers in Scotland, although 94 per cent of the sample accepted that gums could be affected by disease, 71 per cent believed that bleeding gums were normal (Vogan, 1970: 482). There is also much misunderstanding about the prevention of periodontal disorders (Markkula *et al.*, 1977: 112).[2]

The Theory of Focal Infection

In both these instances — controlling tooth decay and assessing the periodontal condition — the state of public information in large part reflects what was until recently the dominant view within the profession itself. This 'culture lag' interpretation receives further support from evidence on the distribution in the population of items of health information; generally speaking, those social strata that are most far-removed from the profession are also those that are likely to be most markedly out of step with the current state of professional opinion on health matters. What the 'culture lag' notion suggests is that the lay culture is a dynamic and changing phenomenon that is shaped by various agencies. Emphasis has been given to the impact on popular opinions of intellectual developments within the dental profession itself; this is partly because this is one area where evidence is available. But other agencies may well be more important. Commercial interests and the mass media, changing life circumstances in the areas of standard of living, educational attainment, access to care, dietary practices and patterns of disease must all exert a major influence in shaping the popular culture of dentistry.

But what the 'culture lag' notion also suggests, apart from the dynamic and changeful nature of the lay culture, is that the beliefs and routines of the dental profession itself are by the same token subject to change and development. If we accept that the profession has been an important influence in determining the changing nature of lay views of oral health and oral care, then we must also be persuaded to regard professional beliefs and practices in much the same light. In other words, we have to view the practice of dentistry within the same cultural framework since, to approach it in any other way, is to attribute to the prevailing 'conventional wisdom' of the profession an objectivity and a scientific rigour that is hard to justify in the light of what we know about the vicissitudes and controversies of dental practice and debate that enliven the intellectual history of dentistry. Viewing dentistry as a culture, albeit a professional rather than a lay one, has certain distinct advantages.

In the first place it allows us to consider the process by which professional beliefs and routines are produced and shaped, a process that might otherwise easily be interpreted as reflecting a natural evolution of scientific ideas. This is not to deny that dentistry, like any other technical profession, has a body of expertise and skills that is constantly refined and supplemented by scientific research and practical experience. There is such a corpus of theory and practice that has developed in a more or less cumulative manner in step with scientific and technical advances achieved by individual practitioners and scientists, research laboratories, commercial interests, etc. In other words, in many ways dentistry appears to conform to the classic model of cumulative development that is supposed to characterise advances in the natural sciences.

Dentistry is also a practical and technical discipline and, as such, has been subject to the normal pressures of various social, economic and political interests. Hence, just as the dental attitudes and behaviour patterns of various social groups tell us much about their contrasting life-circumstances — their access to information and services; the folk memory of dental care received in the past; and the broader patterns of their way of life — so the professional culture speaks of a history of occupational evolution subject to the influence of a range of factors outside those normally considered to affect the path of scientific development.

The theory of focal infection, for example, is eloquent testimony of the impact of external social forces on the development of scientific ideas. According to the theory, which was in vogue for twenty to thirty years, the mouth was held to be an important, possibly *the* most important, portal of entry for bodily infections and disorders of many kinds. A particularly important source of infection was oral sepsis, especially in its extreme form of gross decay and rotting gums. Such dental foci of infection were thought to be involved in a wide range of disorders, especially the diseased condition of joints (Easlick, 1951: 613).

The original, and most powerful, statement of the theory was expounded by William Hunter in 1910 in his denunciation of the excesses of mechanical dentistry. Hunter pointed to the widespread tendency, among American dentists in particular, to construct gold crowns and elaborate bridge work, concealing gross untreated problems of oral sepsis under a facade of dental reconstruction. This practice stemmed from the fact that most dentists were trained almost exclusively in the mechanical and technical arts of dental construction and took pride in their ability to transform unpromising oral conditions into gleaming bridge work or crowns. Therefore, the biological and medical aspects of oral treatment tended to be neglected, a failing that was reflected in the very rudimentary education dentists received in the biological and medical sciences.

According to Hunter, it was this emphasis on the mechanical aspects of dentistry, and the neglect of therapeutic skills, that left so much oral sepsis hidden by bridge work, untreated and acting as a constant source of infection for other disorders. With the crude diagnostic techniques available at the time, and with gross oral sepsis common because of widespread dental neglect, Hunter's thesis was a persuasive one and it came to be widely accepted within the profession. For at least a generation many dentists took these strictures seriously and any sign of oral sepsis was often excuse enough for the wholesale extraction of teeth that might otherwise be completely sound (Burt, 1978: 276). Although the theory lost adherents in the 1940s, it was not until 1951 that the supposed scientific basis of the theory was completely discredited.[3]

It is, of course, possible to account for the rise and fall of the theory of focal infection in terms of the normal swings and roundabouts of intellectual fashion that are certainly not peculiar to dentistry. After all, medicine has had more than its fair share of specious theories, fads and crazes, and many of these have attracted enthusiastic advocacy within the profession itself. Apart from the vagaries of intellectual fashion one has also to consider the purely practical constraints imposed by the limited diagnostic techniques available at the time, the still elementary nature of knowledge about the body and its functioning, inadequate methods of scientific investigation, etc.

While these are all factors that can explain how a theory, now discredited, could ever have gained such widespread acceptance in the first place, they do not really help us to understand why a specific thesis – in this case, the theory of focal infection – should attain such a prominent place in the intellectual history of the profession, and why this intellectual tide should have occurred at precisely the time that it did. It is in order to answer these questions – why focal theory? why the 1920s? – that we have to consider the influence of wider social factors, and especially the rapidly changing position of dentistry in society.

It was during this period that dentistry was undergoing the transition from manual trade to scientific profession, and the rise of focal theory is probably most plausibly interpreted in this context. It is plausible to suggest that the theory obtained such ready acceptance among dentists because it provided the profession with at least a semblance of a scientific and medical rationale for its work, which till then appeared to the public and practitioners alike to have more in common with the mechanical or cosmetic crafts than with scientific medicine (Easlick, 1951: 612). Ironically for a theory that was to be so comprehensively discredited on scientific grounds, among its most enthusiastic advocates were those who wished to see dentistry accepted as a fully-fledged specialty of medicine, the truly scientific parent discipline. A.J. Asgis, for example, was active in the American Stomatological Association in the 1920s; he edited the short-lived 'Review of Clinical Stomatology', and was also involved in the so-called '100 per cent movement' which was active at the time in proselytising the focal infection principle and which advocated, as its name suggests, the wholesale (100 per cent) extraction of teeth where oral sepsis was suspected (Asgis, 1931: 779).

This association between stomatology and focal infection theory was something that went beyond the activities of prominent personalities such as Asgis. It had as its basis a common strategy for the professional and scientific advancement of dentistry. If dentistry were to shake off its origins in the manual trades, then it had to develop those elements, such as modern scientific theory and the association with medicine, that highlighted the more prestigious and dignified aspects of its task. Hence, the idea that dentistry should evolve as a specialty of medicine, and break with its trading origins, was associated with the advocacy of modern scientific theory, such as the germ origins of infectious diseases and the importance of the mouth as a source of infection for disorders in other parts of the body (Blaugh, 1935: 1860-1).

Although there was this apparent tendency for the most enthusiastic advocates of focal infection theory to be those who wished to see a break with the mechanical tradition and a surge towards the scientific dentistry of the future, the theory survived a considerable time. This was because of the support and advocacy it received from the great majority of practitioners, whose everyday 'clinical impressions' — 'a mixture of science and empiricism' as Easlick (1951: 615) termed it — confirmed, at least to their satisfaction, that oral sepsis contributed in a major way to disorders in other parts of the body. Add to this, aspirations for professional status and acceptance in the wider community of scientific medicine, and one begins to understand the reasons for the rise of focal infection theory and for the tenacious hold it maintained for so long in the dental profession.

In the end it was the scientists who finally and conclusively laid the theory to rest and, in so doing, established the scientific credentials of the future dental practice. It is in this sense, therefore, that the case of focal infection theory reaffirms the idea that scientific advance proceeds relatively independently of direct social and political pressures, though the direction it takes and the way its findings are adapted and used will depend on influences that go beyond the boundaries of the scientific community.

The core theoretical understandings of a discipline like dentistry with any scientific pretensions are unlikely to respond to intellectual fashion after the manner of focal theory. If the theory is flawed, empirical anomalies and puzzles inevitably occur and, while these may merely serve to expand and enrich a practitioner's store of 'clinical impressions', as they did in this instance, a scientific model or paradigm cannot long accommodate too many such anomalies before the base theory itself is brought increasingly into disrepute in the wider scientific community (Kuhn, 1962: 62). What the example of the focal infection theory illustrates, therefore, is not that the core scientific understandings of dentistry are subject to wider social influences, but that the directions of research, the wider application of research findings and the subsequent development of routines and philosophies of dental practice and treatment are all shaped by factors outside the scientific community, and largely outside the profession as well. In other words, it is probably safe to assume in our analysis of the occupational culture that as one moves further away from the central research enterprise and moves closer to the application of that knowledge and closer to the development of professional attitudes, beliefs and patterns of practice, so the influence of social circumstances becomes more marked and easier to discern.

Shaping the Professional Culture

One does not have to move very far from the scientific core of dentistry to detect the impact of external factors; in fact, one has to go no further than the standards of technical expertise, the levels of skill with which knowledge is in practice applied by dental providers. In medicine, for example, there is evidence that, while the type and duration of medical school training does affect clinical performance, and does most emphatically shortly after graduation, the influence of educational background from then onwards decreases as other factors come to have a greater impact.[4] One of the most important of these 'other factors' is the effect of work-setting on clinical performance, though the effect of work-setting seems to be less for those who have received longer periods of training (Rhee, 1977: 10).

In dentistry there is also evidence, though of a limited nature, that the practice environment may have an influence on clinical performance that greatly outweighs the effects of dental school background. Silversin *et al.* (1977), in their 1971 study of practising dentists in the UK, found that dental-school background exerted barely any influence on the preventive nature of dental practice. While the study was rather inconclusive, in that it failed to provide any alternative explanation for the variations in preventive behaviour that existed among British dentists, there is evidence that one reason for the lack of any discernible effect of training on performance — a finding that confirms the evidence from medical practice — is the constraints exerted by the circumstances and demands of a busy modern practice.

This receives some support in another article by the same authors in which comparisons were drawn between the teaching of some clinical aspects of endodontics and the corresponding pattern of dental practice outside the teaching environment (Silversin *et al.,* 1975: 78-9). In this study it was reported that, while over 90 per cent of dental students used a rubber dam or cover most of the time during endodontic procedures, this was true for only a tenth of the practitioners in the sample, all of whom had graduated in the preceding 15 years from the same 12 dental schools in which the teaching pattern for the study was established. Much the same result was evident in the use of radiographs during endodontic treatment. While the students routinely took three radiographs — at initial diagnosis, during treatment and on completion — the majority of practitioners took only one or two, tending to drop the radiograph taken during treatment. Again, educational background seemed to have no effect on clinical performance; as before, it is probably the dictates of a busy modern practice that have produced this relaxation of professional standards.

Patterns, and even standards, of treatment may vary quite significantly according to the predominant social composition of clientele, with the higher social strata receiving much more restorative work — especially crown and bridge work (Bailit, 1978: 299) — and lower social strata tending to have teeth extracted and dentures fitted (Sheiham and Hobdell, 1969: 402-3; Schoen, 1975: 177), a pattern that is also reflected in the treatment of black patients in the USA (Moosbruker and Jong, 1969: 727). Dental practices with a predominantly working-class clientele tend to be less well-staffed and equipped (Cussler and Gordon, 1968: 48), and the dentists working in such practices are not so preventively-inclined (Kesel, 1961: 105), and are generally less progressive and less actively involved in the wider affairs of the professional community (O'Shea, 1971 a : 158). Such social patterning is also evident in primary medical care (Tudor Hart, 1972). The emergence of such contrasting philosophies of treatment is not restricted to those practice contexts where the immediate influence of the clientele can be felt, as is the case in primary care. Different treatment philosophies have emerged in various specialist branches of orthodox medicine,[5] even to the extent of shaping quite distinct philosophies in post-graduate medical education.

On a broader canvas it is also clear that, regardless of the impact of specific social factors on the emergence of particular philosophies and schools of thought within the various branches of medicine, the broad pattern and the long-term trend of medical practice is subject to the influence of outside social and economic factors. A case in point is the current emphasis, and continuing trend towards, the greater use of drugs in most standard therapies. The enormous increase in the use of drugs in recent years may in part reflect their growing efficacy and usefulness in medical practice and, to some extent too, a growing expectation among members of the public that a prescription is a normal and accept-able conclusion to a medical consultation (Waldron, 1977: 37).

But apart from these factors, one important influence on levels of drug prescribing has been the activities of the drug companies themselves in promoting the use of their products. One particularly significant development in this area has been the efforts of the major pharma-ceutical companies to co-opt opinion leaders and researchers in the medical profession, as for example in a recent study in Finland (Hemminki and Pesonen, 1977: 501). Clearly, close linkages of this sort are likely to have a profound impact on the direction of medical practice.

In dentistry it is possible to detect similar developments — on a smaller scale, certainly, but accompanied by much the same combina-tion of social and economic pressures. A similar combination of tech-nical advance, public expectation and commercial pressure has fostered the trend first from 'blood-and-vulcanite' to restorative practice and now, one stage further, to elaborate reconstructive work and preventive procedures.[6]

If the core scientific underpinnings of dentistry are least affected by external social and economic factors, it is on the outer reaches of the professional culture — the common understandings about the organisa-tion, delivery and financing of care — that we find the most limited in-fluence of scientific knowledge and the most profound and decisive impact of broader social and political factors. It is in this area that we come closest to the immediate social and political interests of the pro-fession and closer also to the point at which these interests address wider issues of public concern. With the influence of technical and scientific considerations at their weakest and with the more or less overtly political connotations of issues concerning the organisation and delivery of care, it is not surprising that external factors have a major influence on the formation of professional opinion.

Recent work shows quite marked generational differences in attitudes to the use of auxiliaries, with younger dentists and students being far more open to the delegation of work than their seniors (Martens *et al.,* 1971: 2193). Research in the USA on attitudes among physicians to the financing of medical care shows marked differences both between generations and among the different branches of the profession (Goldman, 1974: 181; Colombotos *et al.,* 1975: 385), and one would expect similar, though possibly less marked, variations to occur in the dental profession. Certainly, public opinion in the USA on the issues of 'dental care as a right' and public aid for dental care for children show strong social class and racial differences (Cohen and Fusillo, 1971: 198), and one would expect these differences to be reflected to some extent among dental practitioners along lines of social class and race background, generation, type of practice and mode of employment.[7]

The image we get, therefore, from viewing dentistry as a culture is of an occupational group that is far more diversified and heterogeneous than the concept of 'profession' might otherwise convey. While there is clearly an underlying unity of purpose and philosophy dictated by the demands of dental practice, over and above this central core of beliefs and practices there is considerable room for diversity and for the influence of factors that have their source outside the profession. More importantly, viewing the occupation as a culture allows us to consider the beliefs and routines of dentistry as cultural traits or attributes shaped by outside social and economic forces, though probably such an approach is less applicable in the analysis of the scientific core of dentistry than it is to treatment philosophy and to notions about the organisation and financing of dental care.

Ritual and 'Sacredness'

If this perspective on a professional culture allows us to recognise elements of diversity and change and their linkages with broader social factors, it also still permits us to consider the possibility that professional beliefs and routines may have a symbolic value of their own, and serve certain broader cultural functions, quite apart from their supposed scientific standing. In other words, if we are to take seriously the contention that dentistry can be viewed as a cultural system, then we

have also to be ready to acknowledge that there may be aspects of professional belief and practice that are sustained, not because they make
any demonstrable contribution to the dental well-being of the individual
or the oral health of the community, but solely on account of their
symbolic value and wider social meaning and the broader cultural functions that they may serve. In this way we may be able to make sense of
aspects of dentistry that are otherwise rather puzzling when considered
in the context of the supposedly scientific and rational basis for dental
practice.

One does not have to go any further than the typical encounter between patient and practitioner to detect the ritualistic aspects of dental
practice. On any strict interpretation of the tasks that need to be carried
out in the patient-practitioner encounter, the white coat, the passivity of
the patient, the lack of verbal communication, the overwhelming impression of orderliness, restraint and formality, all seem to be superfluous, if
not directly counter, to the technical requirements of the task in hand.
At least, this appears to be the conclusion of Linn (1967) in his careful
analysis of the typical interaction between dentist and patient in the
dental surgery or office.

Linn approached the analysis of the patient-practitioner relationship
using Nadel's criteria for the analysis of social roles. Following the logic
of Nadel's approach, Linn first identified those attributes of the behaviour of dentist and patient that seemed to be central to the performance
of the task in hand and which, if changed, would completely alter the
nature of the relationship between provider and consumer. According to
this criterion, Linn identified as central attributes of the relationship the
practitioner's authoritative manner and the patient's conformity to the
exercise of that authority. Beyond these central characteristics were
those aspects of behaviour that could be regarded as rather marginal to
the form of the relationship, and beyond these, aspects of the interaction that could be defined as quite peripheral to the relationship. Even
in the case of these peripheral and residual aspects of interaction, Linn
found little modification of role performance in his (admittedly limited)
sample (except in the case of younger patients, who tended to be treated
in a more informal manner by the dentists involved in the study).

According to Nadel's criteria, these peripheral, but highly visible,
aspects of the interaction — passivity, orderliness, restraint, formality,
lack of communication — can all be viewed as more or less superfluous
to carrying out the roles of dentist and patient. Yet they persist; furthermore, they are obviously regarded by both patient and practitioner alike
as normal aspects of the relationship, despite their marginality to the

central task of attending to the dental needs of the client. In these circumstances one can only conclude that, if such aspects of behaviour perform no useful service function, then they probably serve some broader symbolic requirements that go beyond the immediate necessities of the dental task. One plausible interpretation for the persistence of such 'marginal' aspects of the patient-practitioner relationship is that they serve to enhance the scientific and professional authority of the provider, both in direct contact with the client and, more broadly, in the wider society. At the very least, it is probably safe to assume that such attributes would not have persisted had they detracted in any way from the authority of the practitioner, and it is in this sense − if no other − that these more or less symbolic aspects of dental practice serve certain wider social functions.

These 'sacred' or symbolic aspects of the practitioner's task are more clearly evident in the case of medicine where there is sufficient scope in the task of the medical practitioner to permit emphasis on the dramatic, but rarely used, 'life-saving' skills to the virtual exclusion of the humbler and more routine calls of medical practice. It is this failure to consider the preventive, educational and humbler curative functions of medicine − arguably the great bulk of medical practice − that Frankenberg (1974: 420) sees as underlying the more romantic view of the 'sacredness' of the practitioner's role. This picture of the sacred and superior qualities of the medical practitioner, although still current, is much more characteristic of earlier analyses since, with the growing importance of chronic over acute disorders, the sheer statistical weight of the humbler functions of medicine becomes overwhelming, while the opportunities for the more dramatic interventions have correspondingly decreased (Bloom and Wilson, 1972: 329).

It is not just the statistical composition of medical practice that has changed so substantially with the advent of the chronic diseases; the very form of the patient-practitioner relationship itself has been affected by this change. The patient with a chronic condition now presents a rather different pattern of consultation. In particular, in instances where the condition is of some long-standing, the patient will have developed skills in diagnosis and treatment for the condition that are equal to those of the practitioner, and has probably also become quite skilled in the management of the consultation as well (Davis and Horobin, 1977: 207).

This decline in the 'sacredness' of the medical task has a double significance for dentistry. In the first instance, of course, dentistry has never aspired to the more dramatic, life-saving tasks of medicine, and so this element of 'sacredness' has been absent. Secondly, dentistry deals with two classic chronic conditions, both of which provide ample opportunity for the exercise of basic preventive, educational and restorative skills that are not too far removed from the routine functions of medical practice. Yet, despite what are otherwise very congenial conditions for the development of an open, egalitarian relationship between patient and practitioner, the dominant characteristics of interaction between client and provider are those that serve in most respects to underline the authority and social distance of the provider rather than to contribute more directly to what might reasonably be regarded as the central technical tasks of oral care.

Nor can it be said — in defence of this burden of ritual — that the patient-practitioner relationship is something of merely marginal significance in the task of promoting oral health in the community. In one recent study, for example, in which the effects on caries of control of diet, oral hygiene and treatment were assessed for a sample of children and their parents, treatment experience emerged as by far the most important factor, not only at the individual level of analysis, but at the level of the community and family also (Jenny *et al.*, 1974: 563). In fact, it is probably true to say that the quality and nature of a person's relationship with their dentist is a central factor in determining their pattern of utilisation. Whether it be a preventive pattern of visiting for regular dental check-ups,[8] or dental visiting for the relief of pain or other symptoms,[9] the use of dental services has to be seen within the context of a continuing record of contact with individual dentists in the dental system. The pattern of dental service use probably owes as much to the individual's experience of contact with practitioners on previous occasions as it does to any immediate circumstances of need (Stoeckle *et al.*, 1963: 984).

Diagnosis and treatment are not the only services performed, of course. If we also consider the educational and preventive functions of dental practice, the importance of the dentist-patient relationship takes on a further dimension since there is strong evidence that people draw much of their correct health information from contact with providers. In an early study in this area Pratt found that, although the mass media could be important in imparting information, respondents drew their correct knowledge either from their own experiences of ill-health or, to an even greater extent, from the illness experience of friends and relatives (Pratt, 1956: 39-40). In other words, contact with the health care system can be an important source of health information (Rayner and Cohen, 1977 : 78), as well as an influence on future patterns of utilisation.

The important point about this discussion is not so much the fact that there appear to be aspects of the typical encounter between patient and practitioner that have a broader symbolic significance and that serve largely to underline the authority of the provider. Rather, the significant point is that these elements in the relationship appear to have no basis in the technical requirements of the dental task, nor even to advance (rather than hinder) the attainment of certain professional goals that one might reasonably attribute to the dental enterprise; goals such as encouraging the rational utilisation of dental services, imparting information, etc. In fact, in the instance of verbal communication, it might be supposed that the proverbial reticence of medical and dental practitioners might reasonably be expected to greatly hinder, rather than advance, wider health tasks such as education, prevention, self-care and the sensible use of health services.

Linn (1974: 39-41), in a return to the analysis of the dentist-patient relationship, comes to just this conclusion about the typical interaction in the dental surgery or office. In a small follow-up study to his earlier analysis of the dentist-patient relationship, Linn found that nearly two-thirds of those interviewed after treatment had no questions whatsoever regarding any dental matters, even though much the same proportion could recall having received information from their dentist on tooth-brushing. In other words, while some information was imparted by the dentist, it was presented in such a context that the patient was not encouraged to think any more widely about other aspects of the treatment received. Linn, drawing on his earlier study — which revealed the overwhelming nature of the dentist's authority in the surgery — argues that the typical pattern of interaction between patient and practitioner is such that it provides little opportunity to impart information, although this probably varies according to the busyness of the practice and the age of the dentist (Hellman, 1976: 175). Typically, patients retain little of the information (Skogedal and Helöe, 1979).

Other studies in dentistry have confirmed the importance of practice characteristics and of the patient-practitioner relationship. Wan and Yates (1975: 147), for example, found that certain practice characteristics were associated with higher levels of utilisation; those respondents who claimed that their dentist used a high-speed drill, mailed reminders and carried out prophylactic treatments were also likely to visit the dentist more frequently. While it is impossible in such cases to apportion causal priority — which came first, progressive dentist or active client? — it does at least leave open the possibility that those dentists who have a modern, preventive practice attract and encourage high utilisers. Of course, technical competence and progressive dental practice are not the only attributes that might attract or encourage particular patterns of utilisation. Another study confirms that professional ability is only part of the picture when people come to select their 'ideal dentist'; personality may be just as important (McKeithen, 1966), though technical competence is still probably the most important criterion for middle-class parents at least, especially when considering the choice of dentist for their children (Jenny *et al.,* 1973: 220).

The Symbolic Functions of Practice

Many aspects of the typical consultation between patient and dental practitioner do not seem to be strictly entailed by the technical requirements of the task and this seems particularly true of the supreme reticence of the dentist and true also of the apparently superfluous trappings of authority and status. These aspects of the relationship can probably be better understood as a form of ritual, behaviour that persists not because of the contribution it makes to the performance of specific technical tasks, but because of its wider symbolic significance. Viewed alongside other practices in modern medicine such as the widespread use of placebo therapy, those ritualistic aspects of the consulting relationship go some distance to support the thesis that medicine, and dentistry, serve important symbolic functions, quite apart, that is, from the purely technical purposes of dental and medical practice (Comaroff, 1976a: 79).

In fact, there are a number of features of modern medicine that highlight the non-scientific and ritualistic aspects of its practice: the failure to discard a whole range of therapeutic techniques that are either ineffective or quite possibly harmful; the 'optimistic' bias in the ready acceptance of new theories and techniques; and the widespread belief in and use of placebos. All point to the importance of ritual and symbolism in Western medicine (Comaroff, 1978: 250), i.e. the visit to the practitioner and the ritual of consultation, diagnosis and treatment serve certain functions quite apart from the obvious purpose of relieving suffering and returning the individual to normal functioning.

These symbolic functions are probably more clearly defined in the context of a traditional healing role like that of the medical practitioner than they are in the case of dentistry. Comaroff (1978: 247) suggests two such functions which can reasonably be regarded as almost universal features of the healing process: in the first instance, the necessity to make sense for the individual of their distress and of their apparently chaotic illness experience; and, secondly, the need to help the patient reorder the disruption in his social relations. While such functions are obviously more characteristic of medical practice as such, there are clearly elements in dental practice that serve these goals.

In medicine, these ritualistic and non-scientific features of the healing process have been documented in a number of areas of medical practice. In the management of childbirth Lomas (1966) has argued that much that is pursued in the name of medical necessity in fact serves the purposes of ritual and custom, little of which has changed since pre-industrial times. The control of diabetes is another area where medical procedures are adhered to in a spirit of grim determination to 'go through the paces', in the absence of any scientific proof as to their efficacy (T. Williams *et al.,* 1967).[10] Again, use of the placebo exemplifies ritual and faith substituting for demonstrated effectiveness; in 1938, 10 per cent of medical expenditure in the USA was spent on vitamin preparations that were prescribed, wittingly or unwittingly, as placebos, and it has been estimated that 30-40 per cent of drug prescriptions in the 1950s in the USA fell into the placebo category (Shapiro, 1960: 118). The adoption and relinquishment of pharmaceuticals is another example of the influence of customary and non-scientific practices in medicine.[11] The relative ineffectiveness of many widely used medical procedures (Cochrane, 1972) and the questionable impact of medical intervention on the long-term decline in mortality both further serve to highlight the ritualistic nature of much medical practice.

Such widespread evidence of the apparent irrationality of medical practice suggests that the functions served by custom and ritual go beyond the mere reordering of disrupted social relations or making sense of the individual's distress. An important element must surely be the mystique that surrounds professional judgement and the obstacle that this places in the way of the dispassionate and scientific appraisal of current medical techniques. In dentistry this mystique is probably less evident, if only because of the less esoteric nature of the dental task. But, by the same token, it is also possible to argue that the trappings of professional mystique are actually *more* important to the social position of the dentist, precisely because the basis of knowledge and expertise is less esoteric than that of the medical practitioner. It could be argued that in an occupation like dentistry where much of the work is routine and where much of it could, in principle anyway, be delegated to lesser-trained auxiliaries, the aura and mystique of competence and authority are actually more important than they are in medicine, where the practitioner is dealing with a far broader range of health problems many of which may involve issues of life and death.

While there may be some dispute about the significance of these factors in dentistry, and certainly less documentation than there is in the case of medicine, there are obviously parallels in the role of ritual, convention and sheer superstition in much contemporary dental practice. For example, the popular media package that reiterates the importance of oral hygiene, diet control and regular visits to the dentist may have great symbolic value in the public culture of dentistry, but it has only mixed empirical evidence to support it. In fact, there is just as much unsupported mythology as firm scientific evidence in many statements about the efficacy of toothbrushing and toothpaste (Bibby, 1966: 278), the cariogenicity of different foods (Bibby, 1975: 130), about dental visiting and techniques of toothbrushing (Sutton and Sheiham, 1974: 49-52), the frequency of dental utilisation (Boggs and Schwartz, 1975: 652-3), and even about the recommended frequency for toothbrushing (Lang *et al.,* 1973: 404).

Nor is mythology restricted to the popular imagination or to the fringes of dental practice. Even scientific research in dentistry has come under scrutiny. For example, doubt has been expressed about the broader applicability of research produced in animal studies, a point that brings into question the great bulk of research into caries (Allman, 1971: 222-3). In recent years the search for a vaccine has caught the imagination of the scientific community and now absorbs much of the funding in dental research. Yet we are now informed that such a strategy holds little promise (Frostell and Ericsson, 1978: 81), not because of problems of public acceptance — an argument which has never before presented an obstacle to further scientific research — but because of basic theoretical questions about the possibility of developing a vaccine, questions that one might have expected to see resolved at an early stage in the research process. Such is the ritualistic nature of much scientific research in dentistry that, as Mandel (1978) has argued, major advances could take place in our understanding of the etiology of caries without these being reflected in any way in changes in the pattern of practice.[12]

Aside from health education and research there is further evidence of ritualism in the area of treatment where, as in medicine, many accepted procedures are known to be of limited value. In the USA, for example, little change has taken place in caries prevalence among young adults since the 1930s, despite considerable advances in the techniques of preventive dentistry. Although a greater proportion of the population is keeping its teeth, there is not a lot of evidence that this can be attributed to dental advances; the greater retention of teeth is probably due more to education, affluence, changing philosophies of treatment, and fluoride, rather than health education and the continuity and availability of dental treatment (Burt, 1978: 273, 284).

In Britain there is little evidence that the last hundred years of dental practice has, until recently, been associated with any improvement in the retention of teeth; the study by Lennon *et al.* (1974) suggests that, while the rate of tooth loss has declined over this period for those under the age of 35, there has been no change for the older age groups. Regular attendance at a dentist may add five years to the longevity of the natural dentition (P. Holloway, 1975: 28) and it will lead to higher levels of treatment (Jackson, 1973: 386), but it will not reduce the level of DMF (Sheiham, 1977). However, it may well be the case that treatment is more effective in the case of the periodontal condition, as has recently been claimed by Löe (1978: 330), although there is considerable doubt about the long-term effectiveness of major periodontal surgery (Knutson, 1979: 648). Even the humble amalgam-filling has come under scrutiny. Elderton (1976b: 207) claims that about a third of all restorations probably need replacing at any given time and that in many instances the causes of failure can be traced to the way in which the filling was originally placed; this could be true of up to two-thirds of freshly-placed restorations, in most cases the causes of failure being directly under the control of the clinician (Elderton, 1976a).

Conclusion

Enough has been said of the professional culture of dentistry to suggest that there are, as in medicine, important ritualistic and non-scientific elements in the beliefs and routines of dental practice and that to think of dentistry, at least in part, as a culture may make sense in much the same way that one might make sense of the dental attitudes and patterns of behaviour of the lay community. While the mix of science and superstition might be different between lay and professional cultures, nevertheless they have enough in common in this respect to make the comparison a useful and illuminating one.

On the face of it, the cultural approach encourages one to view all medical systems of practice and belief as equally valid, since it is founded on the premise that such systems must be assessed and evaluated not according to any universal standards but within the terms of the culture in which they are placed. The position adopted here has been less radical. It has been to argue that the 'cultural nature' of dental practice and belief does not hold with uniform effect across the spectrum but becomes more marked as one moves away from the scientific heart of the discipline towards those areas, like the organisation and delivery of care, that intermesh with wider social, political and economic interests.

The value of the cultural approach is threefold. In the first place, by highlighting the relativistic and changeful nature of systems of beliefs and practices, it points to potential sources of future change; just as theories in dentistry have evolved and in turn been discarded within recent memory, so we are likely to witness similar intellectual developments in the future. Secondly, it suggests that many aspects of dental practice persist, not because of any supposed contribution that they might make to the well-being of the individual patient or to the oral health of the community at large, but because they serve purely symbolic purposes. Thirdly, the cultural approach allows one to consider the possibility that lay and professional systems of belief and practice share much in common and respond to similar influences in the wider society. Therefore, many of the generalisations that we are willing to make about popular beliefs — about their origins and their rationale — may equally well be applied to the professional culture itself. In this way we may be able to achieve a more dispassionate and scientific assessment of the central practices and beliefs of the profession.

Notes

1. In Dudding's (1960: 392) study of patient reactions to brushing teeth with water, dentifrice or salt and soda, toothpaste was overwhelmingly preferred to cleaning by toothbrush alone, with powder dentifrice a second choice. The dentifrices also appeared to be more effective in preventing the formation of pellicles, probably because of the greater acceptability of paste and powder to the subjects participating in the study.

2. Significant numbers of those interviewed in this study cited drugs and rinses, hard bread and vegetables and vitamins as possible methods for preventing gingivitis.

3. In the series of contributions edited by Easlick (1951) the following conditions were considered in relation to the possible effects of oral sepsis: valvular heart disease, renal disease, ocular disease, dermatosis, arthritis. For none of these conditions was oral sepsis considered to be a significant contributory factor.

4. The Peterson study of general practice in North Carolina cited in Bloom (1965: 171-2).

5. See Freidson (1966-7: 500).

6. Changes in the oral health characteristics of the British adult population are documented by Beal and Dowell (1977: 203). Also, for commercial interests, see

Howard (1976: 12).

7. Certainly there is evidence for the importance of the racial factor in the USA, where, for example, non-white dental graduates appear to be much more likely voluntarily to set-up practice in manpower shortage areas, many of which have predominantly non-white populations (Montoya *et al.*, 1978).

8. Kasl (1974: 437) argues that check-ups are probably better understood within the context of illness activities − even though they are preventive in emphasis − because people rarely visit a practitioner without some sort of symptom experience to relate.

9. Kasl and Cobb (1966: 259) view the utilisation of services as being much more akin to the use and re-use of a patient-practitioner relationship than an initial process of seeking attention.

10. In this study those patients who knew most about the disease were better able to carry out the required therapy, but achieved less control of their condition. In fact, there was no correlation between performance of the prescribed therapy and control of the disorder. Posner (1977) has elaborated on this more recently.

11. Mapes (1977: 620-3), in his small study of British general practitioners, argues that innovatory prescribing was more 'an act of faith' than anything else and that those failing to relinquish old preparations despite warnings of side-effects were less skilled in pharmacology and had a more pastoral approach to their work. The classic study by Coleman *et al.* (1966: 134) shows that adoption of new drugs was related more to interpersonal networks and previous heavy usage than to any scientific appreciation of the merits of the drug.

12. An American biochemist has argued that research in this area raises 'false hopes for solutions to problems for which an insufficient basis of knowledge is available . . . It is based on the "pill concept"; every disease can be cured if the right pill can be found' (cited by Chubin and Studer (1978: 67)).

7 THE CHALLENGE TO THE CLINICAL MODEL

The Ethos of a Clinical Science

Although it is possible to discern ritualistic and non-scientific elements in the professional culture of dentistry, it is actually the association in the public mind of dentistry with the achievements of modern science that goes much of the way to explaining the high status of the profession and its work. With a number of important developments in the late nineteenth century — such as anaesthesia, antiseptics, a workable motor-driven drill — dentistry grew immeasurably in public esteem; dental care not only became safer and less painful, it even appeared in the public mind to become more effective as well. Much the same developments were taking place in medicine, though in neither case were these advances very rapid. Although public acceptance of medical claims to expertise was well ahead of dentistry's, it was as recently as the turn of the century that the average person visiting a medical practitioner had a better than average chance of obtaining some benefit from the encounter. The achievements of the various health professions in the late-nineteenth century, then, should not be exaggerated, despite the major advances made in the laboratory sciences.

If the experience of the theory of focal infection is any guide, it appears that the urge for scientific status outran the necessary apprenticeship. The profession was so eager for the trappings of scientific status that it was tempted to by-pass the time-consuming business of actually establishing a range of well-tested and validated procedures based on scientific research. Nevertheless, important advances had been made and the focal theory of infection can probably, with the benefit of hindsight, be regarded as no more than a false start on the route to further scientific achievements in dentistry. What has emerged in the wake of these achievements is a set of basic assumptions that guides the profession in its work. It is these working axioms of dentistry that span the great intellectual divide between the world of laboratory research and the practical requirements of a personal service profession, a set of working assumptions that, because of their focus in the clinical sciences, can most conveniently be termed 'the clinical model'.

While it is not actually possible to find a coherent and systematic exposition of such a set of assumptions, one can nevertheless discern the

120

outlines of an intellectual framework that underlies the many and varied endeavours of dentistry and that links these activities to the world of modern science. The first, and most fundamental, of these axioms is the assumption that oral disorders are, for all practical purposes, best understood as the outcome of specific disease processes. This assumption is a crucial one and underlies the great bulk of dental research. The assumption is of such importance because of the intellectual guide it provides for the everyday work routines of the dentist. By associating an oral disorder with a specific disease, one automatically maps out a solution to the sort of clinical problems that constantly face the dental practitioner; if there is a determinate disease process, then it can be analysed, its etiology outlined and concrete mechanisms identified for its control and management.

Apart from its role in research, the assumption is also an important one in the professional life of dentistry. In the first place, it associates the endeavours of the practising dentist with those of the putative parent discipline, medicine. Not only does this harness an entire system of healing practice to the dental task; it also, by association, shares the aura of success that attaches itself to the public achievements of medicine. Secondly the disease concept underlies and justifies active intervention; if a disease or dysfunction is present, then the natural implication is that it should be corrected and reversed. This tendency is reflected in the bias towards active intervention shown in medical practice. Scheff (1963: 97-100) argues that professionals are often faced with uncertainty in the course of their routine duties and, in the case of medicine, it is judged preferable to diagnose sickness rather than to risk passing a sick person as well. This is based on the assumption that the risks involved in an incorrect diagnosis are more tolerable than the potential dangers that might follow in the case of untreated disease. If we add to this 'bias towards intervention' the strength of the humanitarian impulse and the laxness of economic controls, it is evident that the disease concept provides a *carte blanche* for active clinical intervention.

The two remaining assumptions that underlie the 'clinical model' can be more briefly outlined, and to some extent they follow from the first as more subsidiary propositions. A second assumption, then, is that the management and correction of oral disorders can be best approached using the techniques of the biomedical sciences. To some extent such an assumption flows naturally from the idea that oral disorders are best viewed as the outcome of specific disease processes; because a disease is naturally identified as a physiological dysfunction of some sort, it logically follows that the correction of such a dysfunction must also be regarded as a task for biomedical science. More than this, however, the intellectual framework provided by the biomedical sciences, like other technical disciplines, lends itself to the application of well-defined and tangible procedures with measurable outcomes. In dentistry the filling of a cavity with amalgam serves this function and in medicine, possibly the prescription of drugs. Indeed, Renaud (1975: 559) has gone so far as to argue that much of the rationale of modern scientific medicine is merely the translation of health needs into discrete, tangible entities that can then more easily be presented as marketable commodities. Aside from this function − which personalises and makes more tangible the management of oral disorders − it has also been argued that the biomedical perspective serves to direct the energies of the professional to issues of technique rather than to wider questions of a more social and political nature. Therefore, while the disease concept encourages a 'bias towards intervention' in medicine and dentistry, it is the influence of the biomedical sciences that translates the force of this activist philosophy into manageable service packages that can be delivered in a reasonably short space of time in exchange between client and practitioner.

The third, and final, axiom that underlies the 'clinical model' is the assumption that there exists a body of knowledge and expertise about oral disorders and their management and that this corpus of theory provides a relatively objective and clear-cut guide to the routines of dental practice. To some extent this assumption flows naturally from the first two since, if it could not be assumed that there was some objectivity in the application of theoretical knowledge, much biomedical research would lose its rationale and much dental practice its scientific justification. Therefore, the assumption that research can be applied relatively objectively in the daily routines of professional practice is an essential link in the profession's claims to a special competence to deal with oral health. By the same token, it is also the all-important reason why the public tend to accept the profession's claims to exercise a uniformly high level of expertise in routine dental practice. It is in this sense that the assumption of objectivity is the most important of all, since it provides the all-important basis for the high level of public confidence that the health professions enjoy.

Although the puzzles and anomalies that have arisen within dentistry are many and varied, it is possible to discern four broad areas of concern where the failings of the clinical model have been particularly striking. In the first place, it has become increasingly clear that the ruling assumptions of professional dentistry about appropriate treatment and about the rational use of dental services are not necessarily accepted in the population at large and, indeed, may vary greatly in their acceptance between different social groups. While much of the theory of dental practice is based on certain premises about the desirability of preserving the natural dentition and about regular visits to the dentist for maintenance care, this philosophy finds few adherents outside those strata that lie closest to the dental profession, predominantly the middle and upper reaches of the middle class. Secondly, the assumptions of objectivity that underlie the disease concept do not reconcile with popular conceptions of dentistry that associate it more with cosmetics than with health; this is most obviously the case with orthodontics, but it is also true in other areas of dental practice. Also, in many areas genuine alternative philosophies of dental treatment exist, ranging from a pragmatic repair and extraction service at one extreme to elaborate restorative work at the other. Such variety of treatment philosophies, together with the cosmetic associations of dental care, do much to undermine the claims to objectivity based on the disease concept of oral health need.

Thirdly, under conditions of normal dental practice, the type of treatment provided to the client is affected just as much by social and economic factors as it is by any standards of scientific appraisal. This follows logically enough from the first two generalisations. If prevailing professional concepts of treatment and service use are not widely accepted in the population, and if the disease concept of oral health need does not provide an unequivocal guide for clinical intervention in dental practice, then it seems natural enough that non-clinical considerations will often prevail. This is epitomised in the case of the extraction of teeth where, in the case of the lower socio-economic strata at least, social and economic factors tend to override purely clinical criteria. Finally, despite the supposed unity of theory and practice in clinical dentistry, in reality widely varying treatment philosophies have emerged under different conditions, reflecting the influence of contrasting national traditions and responding to the immediate pressures of dental practice. Yet, while there *is* this variety in the delivery of care, the dominant professional ideal remains that of technically proficient restorative dentistry, an 'ideal' that governs the content and goals of dental education and that guides the policies of the profession.

Elements of Subjectivity

The critical nature of the situation is clearly evident in orthodontics where shortcomings in the clinical model are most apparent, shortcomings that are largely due to the attempt to impose professional notions of the faulty alignment of mouth and jaws (malocclusion) *as a disease,* onto popular conceptions that associate malocclusion with personal appearance and aesthetics. In case it should be thought that the issue arises merely from a clash of perspectives between the profession and the public, there is also evidence of considerable diversity even within the profession itself. For example, in a recent review of the literature carried out by Jago (1974: 82), it has been established that the rate of malocclusion, as assessed in 94 professional field surveys, can vary anywhere between one and 90 per cent for populations studied in 18 different countries. It is, of course, possible that such variations may be due to 'real' differences in the prevalence of malocclusion. Also, part of the explanation for such discrepancies may be the differing degrees of handicap qualifying for inclusion in the studies reviewed by Jago. More likely still, such variations reflect a lack of agreement between investigators in assessing the orthodontic handicap, a lack of consensus that exists even in professional ratings of the most extreme cases of malocclusion. Draker (1970: 136-8), for example, found in his study on rating dental casts for physical handicap that there was complete agreement among the raters on less than 40 per cent of the casts and that, on repeating the task after a period of 24 hours, 15-20 per cent of the previous judgements were reversed.

But apart from this apparent variation in professional judgements of 'need', which may only be a question of ensuring greater comparability in the indices used in different studies, there is also the fact that the clinical definition of need, which is based on the disease analogy, is one that rarely coincides with consumer definitions. Indeed, as Friedman (1971: 63) has pointed out, the disease analogy is itself flawed in that the standard by which orthodontic need is judged – the normal or ideal occlusion – is so rarely encountered that it is itself quite an abnormal condition. In other words, orthodontic handicap is assessed in terms of departures from some theoretical ideal occlusion, rather than by any objective definition of handicap or some other abnormality. Furthermore, most treatment is carried out for cosmetic reasons rather than for any health purpose, and the subjectivity of orthodontics is entirely apparent.

The consumer reaction in this area underlines the point. In a number of studies it is clear that a very small percentage of those with clinically defined orthodontic handicap are in fact interested in undergoing corrective treatment. For example, in the study by Ingervall *et al.* (1978), although 76 per cent were assessed as needing treatment, and a third were aware of this, only 2 per cent actually wanted treatment. In Myrberg and Thilander's (1973) study of school children, a higher proportion – between a half and three-quarters of those in need – were 'interested' in treatment. This is not to say that there is necessarily any great diversity in popular notions of the 'acceptable' or 'desirable' shape of teeth and jaws, at least in countries of a European cultural tradition. Cohen's (1970: 648) work in the USA, for example, suggests that much the same standards of personal appearance are held by members of very different social groups. But, while aesthetic standards may appear to be much the same, it is the demand for treatment that varies. It is generally the middle class who make heavier demands on orthodontic services (Kegeles, 1974a: 121), whether because of economic factors, greater concern with personal appearance, or provider influences, is not clear.

In work carried out on patient assessments of treatment need, there is undoubtedly some correspondence with provider judgements based on standard, objective indices of need (Katz, 1978: 333), although even for the 'best' of the professional indices – Angle's classification – the relationship with patients' satisfaction with their appearance is weak. The Treatment Priorities Index is another measure that correlates with popular assessments of orthodontic treatment need, especially at the extremes of the spectrum of need (USPHS, 1973; 1977). Nevertheless, despite this correspondence between professional and client definitions of need, until criteria of cosmetics and personal comfort govern the construction of such indices, rather than some notional concept of perfect health, marked discrepancies in the assessment of the orthodontic handicap will remain. Such is the magnitude and extent of these discrepancies that they raise wider questions about the viability of the framework from which the concept of orthodontic need is derived. But aside from this conceptual or philosophical challenge to the clinical model, there are also economic factors to consider. Apart from anything else, the commitment of resources to orthodontics that would in principle be required if the disease analogy were to be followed, would be quite out of proportion to any conceivable social benefit. With the evidence that orthodontic coverage is increasingly being written into labour union contracts in the USA, this is no longer an academic question (Jenny, 1975). In principle, there is no reason why economic considerations cannot be accommodated in orthodontic assessments. It would, of course, require a frank appraisal of the limitations of the clinical model; but, at the same time, it would probably salvage the scientific status of orthodontic treatment. Recent research on the determination of orthodontic needs in the light of limited resources has shown that some objectivity can be attained in this matter (Grewe and Hagan, 1972: 293-4).

Need and Demand

It is in these two respects — the economic implications of taking the disease analogy seriously and the public image of dentistry as being concerned more with cosmetics and personal comfort than with health — that the disease concept of oral disorder fails to take account of wider social factors. While the discrepancy is particularly striking in the case of orthodontics, the point applies with equal force to caries and to periodontal disease. Both are conditions that conform more closely than orthodontics to public conceptions of ill-health and disease, but neither equates well with more widely accepted concepts of health (Kelman, 1975: 630). If, for example, we take health as being freedom from illness then, as in the case of orthodontics, this commits us to radical and wide-ranging programmes of prevention and treatment, programmes that it would not be possible to justify on economic or social grounds considering the minimal health importance of the conditions involved. If, on the other hand, we adopt a more pragmatic, functional definition of health gauged according to the individual's ability to carry out certain key social roles, then such a measure would direct us to very minor programmes of intervention, because it would be insufficiently sensitive to pick up either caries or periodontal disease, except in their most extreme and advanced forms.

In fact, on this definition, oral health problems can only be classified along with other minor conditions of personal comfort and cosmetics such as obesity and baldness, conditions which can scarcely be considered matters of national concern (Cohen and Jago, 1976: 694). If, with Fanshel (1972: 320), we consider health and well-being to reflect the extent to which a person is able to carry out his usual daily activities, then oral disorders barely feature in any significant way. On any continuum of dysfunction or disability, oral disorders are closer to the categories of discomfort and dissatisfaction, neither of which involve any significant limitation on normal activities. Only the most extreme and rarest cases even enter the category of 'minor disability', a fact that is borne out by research showing that, while in principle people regard dental problems as sufficiently serious to warrant exemption from normal activities, in practice this is less likely to be observed (Gerson, 1972).

Like other chronic disorders such as diabetes, the oral disorders may not involve major disability and symptom-related visits, but they can involve a lifetime's commitment to treatment and a life-long contact with providers of care. Chronic disorders of this kind require a rather special relationship between client and practitioner since the motivation for treatment and self-care is not supported by the usual symptoms of illness. With chronic conditions of this kind, people are not usually regarded as sick, and so the basis for their relationship with the practitioner is not one of patient/healer — which naturally favours the status and authority of the practitioner — but client/consultant, which introduces a degree of equality and mutual respect and co-operation into the relationship (Bloom and Wilson, 1972: 324). But, if there is this similarity in principle in the patient-practitioner relationship, there is also the difference that, unlike the case of diabetes, failure to control oral disease may not have serious consequences for the individual's ability to live a normal life. Therefore, while individuals must in the case of oral health problems enter the dental care system as patients from time to time, they do not in any way regard themselves as disabled or sick in so doing, unlike the circumstances of most other chronic health conditions.[1] The only way in which, dental utilisation overlaps with other health concerns is in the extent to which, as with other chronic conditions, a visit to a practitioner may be seen, not as curing a condition — which may apply in the case of acute problems — but as halting its further deterioration (Parsons, 1975: 259).

If oral health problems, therefore, have little to do with a person's ability to carry out their usual daily activities, they probably have much more to do with the individual's quality of life and personal comfort (Giddon, 1978). While there is evidence that dental satisfaction may bear little relation to any clinical assessment of the oral condition in the case of those with their own natural teeth (the dentate) (Barenthin, 1977: 73), for those *without* natural teeth (the edentulous) there is a fairly close relationship between satisfaction and the ability to use dentures (Seifert *et al.*, 1962: 522). Among the elderly in particular, the ability to use dentures satisfactorily is likely to be especially important, as much for their mental and emotional well-being as for their physical health (Ettinger, 1973: 19). For the dentate, the fact that only a fraction of those with oral problems actually visit a dentist[2] means, as in the case of medical services, that the dental system is rescued from the consequences of having adopted a treatment-orientation based on a simple disease concept of oral health need. The fact is that, were more than a fraction of the actual clinically defined need in the population to be translated into effective demand for services, the dental system would be overwhelmed. It is only because of the enormous gap between need and effective demand that the restorative philosophy (P. Holloway, 1975: 29) has survived with any scientific credibility at all.

The philosophy rests on the assumption that, if patients can be reached on a regular basis, the treatment that they receive can halt irreparable damage and loss of function. The philosophy has validity as long as attention is restricted to those willing and able to visit the dentist on a regular basis. To this extent it has provided perfect justification for the practice of dentistry as a private contract between a dentist and a patient willing or able to pay a fee. But once we widen our vision beyond regular, fee-paying attenders to the population as a whole, the theory loses much of its impact, in large part because of the enormity of the task that presents itself. In the induction of men in the American army during the Second World War, for example, dental defects were the single major cause of rejection prior to Pearl Harbour (Goldstein, 1951: 605). Once the commitment had been made after Pearl Harbour to attempt to rehabilitate those with recoverable deficiencies, over a million bridges and dentures were fitted and 31 million cavities filled — and this for a group that one could reasonably expect to be above average in physical condition for the active age groups in the population, not counting those who were too old for military service and therefore likely to be in greater need of care.

If the example of the American mobilisation is any guide, the commitment of resources required for full treatment-coverage in any given adult population is likely to be enormous, as some Nordic countries are now beginning to discover.[3] Even were it possible to provide full treatment coverage for a population, there is still no guarantee that prolonged dental treatment can postpone tooth loss for anything more than five years (P.J. Holloway, 1975: 28), nor is there any guarantee that such benefits can survive a long-term break in the continuity of service.[4] The same reasoning applies just as much in the case of periodontal disease as it does for traditional, conservative treatment. The option of running a treatment-oriented system is just as limited since, according to current WHO (1978: 24) estimates, a dentist can only provide a full annual periodontal service for 400-500 patients, a figure that leaves any realistic manpower projections far short of the potential demand.

There is, then, an extraordinary imbalance between resources and potential demand in a treatment-oriented system — whether this be in the instance of orthodontic services, or conservative treatment, or periodontal care. In the absence of any explicit rationing of services under these conditions, the market and various barriers to care apportion dental health resources in the population. The fact, for example, that 10 per cent of the American population absorbs 75 per cent of dental resources[5] speaks both to the rationing function of the price mechanism in the free market and to the enormous potential expenditure of resources that would follow if similar facilities and standards of care were to be provided for the whole population. Recently, the question of rationing has been more squarely faced, at least in academic circles.[6] In the health area some have argued for the application of minimum standards of personal health service (Rosenthal and Fox, 1978: 1), preferring a universally achieved minimum to a theoretical or ideal perfection that is unattainable and that, in any case, serves in the main to obscure the inegalitarian tendencies of current rationing systems. In the case of dentistry Barenthin (1975: 47) has argued that, in the absence of effective prevention, we should be setting flexible and realistically attainable goals in the provision of dental services. This may mean that, for those communities where resources are limited and the backlog of need considerable, dental services will have to be restricted, in the preliminary stages at least, to the relief of pain and to ensuring only that certain minimum standards of dental health are met in the population at large. WHO (1965; 1976) has recognised this and published guidelines for administrators and policy-makers to establish priorities in treatment planning and population coverage.

The Social and Economic Context

This is a second area, therefore, where the clinical model is clearly deficient. Aside from issues of subjectivity and the inaptness of the disease analogy, it is also clear that the clinical model has not accommodated the effects of the economic and social factors that have been detected in medical practice. Without such adjustments to the model it cannot aspire to provide an adequate guide to what actually happens in the daily round of dental practice. As a set of axioms that underlies the work of dental educationists and researchers and that informs both the self-image and the public view of the profession, the clinical model is based on the assumption that there exists a body of knowledge and techniques in dentistry that can be applied to most oral health problems in a relatively scientific and objective manner. Yet, one does not have to look far to see that the application of this body of theory is, in the real world, influenced by a range of social and economic factors.

The closest parallels in medical practice are surgery and the prescription of pharmaceuticals or drugs. Surgery is a close parallel because, like much dental work, operations can be regarded as discrete, quantifiable packages of service that also have highly visible results. Also, for procedures like tonsillectomy, varicose-vein-stripping, hemorrhoidectomy, elective hysterectomy and cholecystectomy, surgical operations approximate the very discretionary character of most dental interventions. It is in such areas of surgical practice that, because of their elective nature, operations are especially sensitive to the availability of resources (Vayda, 1977).

The prescription of pharmaceuticals is also an area where a clear parallel with dental practice can be drawn. It is here that one can discern, more clearly than in most areas of medical practice, the pressures exerted on the practitioner by the constraints of time, patient demand, the activities of commercial interests, and even by the practitioner's own self-image as the efficacious provider of care. At the most basic level, the pressure on medical practitioners follows directly from the expectation — held on both sides of the desk — that, within the brief interval of the average consultation, they will be able to provide a reasonably satisfactory resolution to patients' complaints. A drug prescription is a particularly tangible — and highly symbolic — evidence that such an effective outcome to the consultation has been achieved. Taking into account the practitioner's characteristic 'bias towards intervention' (Scheff, 1963: 99), patient expectations that a prescription will be provided and the practitioner's perception of those expectations,[7] it then comes as a surprise to learn that a prescription is *not* an automatic outcome of the average consultation.

The point here is not so much that prescriptions are a frequent outcome of the average consultation, but that in many cases such an outcome reflects not the legitimate demands of therapy but the effects of extraneous social and economic pressures. In fact, Freidson (1960: 380) goes so far as to argue that the prescription of placebos — which is what we are really talking about when we say that the legitimate demands of therapy are not being met — could be used as a reasonable index of medical practitioners' susceptibility to the demands of their practice clientele. Where clients are referred by other practitioners, or where market conditions are such as to remove the need to compete strenuously for custom, the prescription of placebos will be lower than in those circumstances where practitioners feel that they have to yield to client demands — or what they see as being client demands — for pharmaceutical prescriptions.[8]

The availability of resources and the changing nature of technology and standards of practice place very broad limitations and constraints on the professional enterprise. Andersen and Newman (1973: 103-5) maintain that the increase in the USA in the gross measures of health service use over the last 40 years has much to do with the changing pattern of technology — for example, drugs, anaesthetics, surgery — as well as changing social and professional standards about hospitalisation, the appropriate use of technology, financing care, etc.

In the case of dentistry, the distribution of manpower and other resources may well continue to shape the uptake of dental services in the population, even at the same time as improvements in productivity are increasing the volume of care that is available. In the USA, although no change has taken place in the population: dentist ratio over the last 25 years, there has been a 50 per cent increase over this same period in the number of people seeing the dentist and a 25 per cent increase in the number of visits. In principle there is no reason why such dramatic improvements in productivity should not widen the uptake of dental services and lead to a more equitable matching of resources and health needs. But, as Leverett (1975) has pointed out, in the absence of any redistribution of manpower and other resources, such increases in productivity and the likely future deployment of auxiliaries, far from alleviating existing disparities, are likely to maintain, if not actually to reinforce, them. Further evidence of the constraining influence of the distribution of resources comes from the UK in a recent article by O'Mullane and Robinson (1977) who show that in an area where the dentist-to-population ratio is more favourable, not only is there a higher uptake of dental services, but there is also evidence that social-class discrepancies in treatment and use of services are significantly reduced.

Organisational Constraints in Dental Practice

The availability of resources, therefore, plays an all-important role in shaping the level of professional intervention and the extent to which these services are distributed among different groups in the population. It also influences the form that such services can take. What this means is that, in the absence of any conscious change in the direction of current manpower policies, the increase in the numbers of auxiliaries being trained is likely to lead to an intensification of present patterns of practice rather than to their substantial modification. In part such an emphasis on the treatment task may reflect public expectations, though evidence in medicine on patient expectations regarding the prescription of drugs suggests that pressure of this sort can easily be overrated. The emphasis on the treatment task is probably due in the main to the core requirements of professional practice. In essence, the fundamental requirement is that, in the brief interval of a professional consultation, some tangible resolution of the client's problem or problems is achieved. A further desirable feature is that the service which is provided should take the form of some discrete, visible and quantifiable item that can be the basis both for the remuneration of the practitioner and for the satisfaction of the consumer's need to feel that something concrete has been done on his behalf.

In third-party payment systems this tendency is, if anything, even more marked since watchful paymasters require fairly tangible evidence that services claimed for have in fact been carried out. Nippert (1978: 9-13), for example, talking in the context of the German health insurance system, argues that while there are preventive measures available that could be implemented in dental practice, they cannot be applied under the prevailing system because of the economic bias towards tangible and quantifiable restorative treatment, a bias that is strongly reinforced by the pressure of patient expectation. One item of service that qualifies particularly well under this rubric is prosthetic treatment, which can be among the most lucrative items of dental practice (A. Hamilton, 1963: 377), probably because, like other treatment services, it is more of a manufactured item than a service as such and so can be costed and priced accordingly.[9] Crown and bridge work is another. In a study of insurance-plan patients Bailit *et al.* (1979: 702) found that although only 10 per cent of the sample had received crown and bridge work, this accounted for a third of programme costs. Even patient-oriented preventive procedures can be made remunerative, again especially where the element of manufacture is enhanced at the expense of the service component (Howard, 1976: 12).

Within the broad boundaries dictated by the availability of resources and the form of the delivery system, practice characteristics play an important part in shaping the volume and pattern of service delivery. In medical practice, for example, even the quality of services has been shown to be affected by the organisational setting in which care is provided. So, in Rhee's (1976) study, large group practices provided higher quality care than solo settings, though there was no discernible difference between solo and smaller group practices. Different methods of paying medical practitioners may also have some effect on various aspects of the delivery of services such as health status, continuity of care, access, the comprehensiveness of services provided, the personal nature of care and the efficiency of service delivery (Boudreau and Rivard, 1976: 61-2). In particular, it is probably true to say that, because of the incentive to service involved, insurance schemes generate a greater volume of professional services than do pre-paid plans (Faltermeyer, 1970: 126), which, in turn, tend to encourage a more efficient use of medical resources (Pineault, 1976: 135). It has also been suggested that a reduction in the direct price barrier in pre-paid plans contributes to more aggressive consumer behaviour; clients may feel that they have a contractual right to service and the practitioner is unable to use the fee-barrier as a means of curtailing consumer demand (Freidson, 1973a: 473).

In dentistry there is evidence that capitation schemes may improve the preventive style of practice, reduce the number of fillings placed and produce a more favourable dental health outcome (Rosen *et al,* 1977: 228). The financial savings introduced by such schemes are modest, however (Bailit *et al,* 1979). Aside from payment, another variable is that of manpower structure. It is possible to experiment successfully with alternative manpower configurations since much of the routine work of the graduate dentist can be performed by a trained auxiliary without loss of quality (Roder, 1973: 319), and with considerable savings in cost (Hankin, 1977: 223). There are also substantial economies of scale to be gained by adding just one dentist to a solo practice, though the gains taper-off after that (BDA, 1976). Alternatives to private funding are also feasible since the conventional wisdom that publicly funded systems of delivering care are inherently less efficient than private practice is not supported by recent research in the USA (Doherty and Vivian, 1976: 8; Doherty, 1978: 519). In fact, on the contrary, there is evidence in the USA that private practice tends to be more costly because of excessive charges of 10 to 20 per cent that have to be paid by the consumer in excess profit (Doherty and Horowitz, 1979).

As in the case of medical practice, therefore, aspects of the delivery system and broad social and economic factors exert their effects on the volume, pattern and type of dental service being provided; yet this finds little place in professional thinking about dentistry. Acccording to the clinical model — as it is taught in dental schools and as it is observed and honoured in the public utterances of leaders of the profession — there exists a body of knowledge and techniques that can be applied in dental practice in a relatively scientific and objective manner. Yet, as is clear from research in medicine, social, organisational and economic factors are crucial in determining the volume and pattern of professional intervention. In dentistry, there is similar evidence in the case of the extraction of teeth, preventive procedures, orthodontics, in fact for the entire range of available dental procedures. This is not to say that such departures from the strict application of clinical acumen are in some way 'wrong' or 'unprofessional', but merely that in the simplicity of its assumptions — assumptions based on a simple translation of biomedical theory out of the laboratory and into dental practice — the clinical model provides a poor guide to the understanding of what goes on in the everyday practice of dentistry.

Conclusion

The implications of this would not be so drastic were it not for the fact that the clinical model has come to dominate not only the research enterprise — which is its intellectual inspiration and source — but also the thinking of the public and the profession and, most importantly, the formulation of policies in the dental area. In this respect dentistry is no different from any other profession in its drive to structure our thinking and to dominate policy initiatives in its own area of concern. McKinlay (1973: 77), for example, has argued that dominant occupations, like the professions, are in a uniquely powerful position to initiate, direct and regulate widespread change. Therefore, we should not be surprised if such social change as does occur in an occupational area will be directed in such a way as to be largely consistent with the interests of the profession concerned.

In dentistry it is the clinical model that reigns supreme and, with it, an entire view of the dental task as being one that is almost wholly accommodated in the world of the biological sciences. The appreciation of social factors is scarcely allowed for within prevailing notions of dental practice. In the USA, for example, arguments for the place of preventive and community dentistry in dental education were made as early as 1918 by the Dental Education Council and a recommendation that 5 per cent of curriculum time should be allocated to these subjects was made in 1934 by the Curriculum Survey Committee. Yet, these very modest recommendations were never implemented by the average dental school (Petterson and Littleton, 1971: 260). As late as 1968-9, this bare minimum had still not been achieved, and in the 47 dental schools surveyed by Petterson the amount of time devoted to the social sciences was a derisory 0.7 per cent (Petterson and Littleton, 1971: 260). It is even possible that what little time *is* being spent on these subjects in dental school actually works to counter any interest in public health issues. According to a study at the University of Alabama, the longer students remained at dental school, the less favourable their attitudes on public health issues became (Ramirez *et al.,* 1967: 527). The position in the research field is no better. At the 1978 conference of the International Association of Dental Research (IADR), of over 1,000 papers presented, less than 10 per cent had any social science content at all (IADR, 1979).[10]

If, as has been claimed, thinking in the oral health field *has* been so entirely dominated by the clinical ethos, then how would a model influenced by the social sciences differ in any substantial way? Table 7.1 spells out some of the main ways in which a model inspired by the social sciences would differ from the dominant mode of thinking in dentistry. In the first place, a far more pragmatic criterion of oral health would displace the current reliance on the disease analogy.

Table 7.1: Conceptual Model

	Clinical	Social
Definition of need	Based on disease analogy	Based on criteria of impairment and disability
Crucial point of intervention	Diagnosis of a condition	Contact with delivery system
Service outcome	Clearly entailed by diagnosis	Strongly affected by non-clinical factors

Secondly, much greater recognition would be given to the role of the delivery system itself in uncovering and determining need and in translating need into effective demand. Thirdly, full recognition would be given to the role of non-clinical factors in determining service outcomes.

Such a model has implications for our understanding of the dental system at the level of individual behaviour — the interaction between patient and practitioner, for example — and at the level of policy formation and institutional change. At the level of individual action it is possible to argue that the social model provides a far closer approximation to the way in which people think about their health and get to see a dentist, and how eventual treatment outcome is determined. The policy implications of the social model are far-reaching. In the first place, in adopting a more pragmatic criterion of oral health we are able to establish social and economic priorities of intervention that permit us to narrow down the otherwise virtually unlimited pool of dental need in the population. Under such an approach it is possible to say that some dental needs are more pressing than others (for example, relief of pain over cosmetics), some social groups should take precedence over others (for example, children over those who have mastered self-care), and certain types of intervention will be more cost-effective than others (water fluoridation over full treatment-coverage). In default of such explicit setting of priorities an alternative, and implicit, rationing system has established itself, one that on most counts fails to meet demonstrated social needs.

Secondly, in recognition of the role that non-clinical factors — including the delivery system — play in shaping service outcomes, far closer attention would have to be paid to the way in which resources are allocated (for example, the geographic distribution of manpower), and to questions of access, and the operation of incentive systems and organisational factors in determining the direction and impact of the delivery system. Again, by default such factors have been allowed to shape the dental system in ways and in directions that do not necessarily meet the needs of the population it ostensibly serves.

Notes

1. This distinction draws on Frankenberg's (1974: 418-19) argument that prevailing notions of service utilisation fail to distinguish between sickness and patienthood. By extrapolation, it could be argued that users of dental services become patients on entering the system, but at no time consider themselves to be sick or in ill-health. The person with a chronic health problem such as diabetes enters the medical system from time to time, but, by contrast to the dental user, acknowledges that there is something wrong which will harm their health if they do not control it.

2. A recent Finnish study found that only a third of those suffering from toothache had visited a dentist (Rajala *et al.*, 1978: 121).

3. For the case of Norway, see Burt (1974). More recent evidence from the USA confirms the enormity of the task, with two-thirds of the population requir-

ing dental treatment of some sort, much of this being simple treatment of decay (USPHS, 1979).

4. Recent research on the Finnish school dental service suggests that the high treatment levels that it attains for those in its care do not provide any long-term advantage (Ainamo and Holmberg, 1973: 30). Danish research suggests, on the other hand, that the school experience may have a levelling effect on oral health differences between social strata (Antoft *et al.*, 1974: 305).

5. See note 9, Chapter 5.

6. With the more stringent economic circumstances of the 1970s, there is now a much more explicit recognition of the fact that services have to be rationed where, as is always the case, resources are scarce (Judge, 1978: 1-4). Also, see M. Cooper (1975).

7. Comaroff (1976a: 90-1) argues that practitioners actually tend to over-estimate client expectations in this regard. While practitioners tend to claim that they are merely responding to patient demand for drugs, among Comaroff's study patients only 51 per cent said that they expected to get a prescription.

8. Nor are such patterns necessarily restricted to medical practice. Elliott (1972: 118-20), for example, cites evidence to show that just such pressures to accede to the client exist in solo legal practices serving ethnic minority and working-class clienteles. Such patterns have also to be understood in the context of the limited amount of time available in which to assess the client's problem. Given the pressure of time, practitioners come to rely on a limited range of diagnoses that 'fit' the normal spread of clients' problems. The operation of such a mechanism has been discussed by Scheff (1966) in the context of rehabilitation agencies, and by Sudnow (1965) for court proceedings.

9. In her analysis of the impact of dental insurance on the pattern of utilisation in Sweden, Barenthin (1976: 215) found that the only increase in treatment received was in the area of prosthetics, which confirms the experience in Britain at the start of the NHS when there was an avalanche of pent-up demand for dentures.

10. Of these, a third were in epidemiology (biostatistics, genetics and public health), which leaves only about 70 papers out of a total of over 1,300 — about 5 per cent — in mainstream social science research in dentistry.

8 FUTURE DIRECTIONS IN DENTISTRY

The neglect of the social sciences and of public health issues is sympto-matic of a far more fundamental flaw in the intellectual framework of contemporary dentistry. This central conceptual fault – in dentistry as in medicine – is that the clinician's focus remains the mechanism of disease rather than its etiology (Payne, 1965: 402).[1] In one sense this focus of concern is entirely understandable. Our knowledge of etio-logical processes is far more limited than our understanding of the pro-gress of diseases and how to manage them and so the choice of direc-tion seems a natural one. Therefore, to say that there is a central con-ceptual fault is not to imply that there is anything inherently wrong in the clinical approach. Once it is allowed to dominate thinking, however, not only in the research laboratory but in the field of policy initiative, it has a severely limiting effect on the range of potential policy options that can be considered and it handicaps our thinking about the applica-tion of a great range of possible avenues of intervention.

Indeed, it can be argued that the apparent simplicity and greater tractability of disease processes – over questions of etiology – are entirely illusory. Robertson (1975: 169) maintains, for example, that the acute, infectious diseases of an earlier age were in principle no more susceptible to thinking in terms of simple causality and specific intervention than the chronic disorders of the twentieth century. These conditions were acknowledged at the time to be just as heavily implicated in a complex and multiple causality. The secret of past successes in this area, accord-ing to Robertson, was not the identification of a simple causal chain of disease etiology but the discovery of certain crucial points of interven-tion that could be manipulated and that could be controlled in such a way as to prevent human damage. It is possible, of course, that the general health area lends itself better to such intellectual clarity because the impact of broader factors, and thus the potential for intervention, is more easily conceptualised. This advantage lies simply with the direct, measurable impact of disease on the individual's ability to perform cer-tain key social roles. Because of this simple property, the effects of death and disease can easily be charted. For example, there is the impact on economic production that can clearly be measured and that can equally clearly be linked to specific environmental factors.[2] In principle, there is no reason why a similar methodology could not be applied in

138

the case of oral health, though, because oral disorders rarely affect an individual's social capacities, there is less incentive than there is in the case of general health to introduce preventive measures.

The Institutional Framework

The search, then, should be for points of intervention, rather than for a definitive social etiology. In this context, perhaps the most distinctive contribution of the social analysis of dentistry is the emphasis on institutional rather than individual forms of health intervention. At first sight it might appear rather difficult to imagine forms of intervention that do not involve identifying and isolating avenues for individual action and initiative, but one does not have to look much further than the rise of organised dentistry itself to identify a number of important social institutions that are deeply implicated in issues of oral health and oral care and that therefore offer themselves as obvious candidates for inclusion in such a scheme. These are, organised dentistry itself, the dental supply industry and what one sociologist has called 'the manufacturers of illness' (McKinlay, 1974) which, in the case of dentistry, must refer to the sugar lobby and the food industry generally. Together with an understanding of the social structure and major cultural features of the advanced industrial societies, these three institutional areas provide a framework for the social analysis of oral health care.

Perhaps the area of most immediate interest because of its impact and because of the potential for policy intervention is what McKinlay has called 'the manufacturers of illness'. By this term McKinlay means to refer to those institutions which, in the course of their routine social functioning, actually create and maintain health risks at levels beyond those associated with the normal variety and hazards of life. These risks to health are 'surplus' to, or above and beyond, that level of personal hazard that is inescapable if people are to lead reasonably varied and interesting lives. In other words, they are those hazards which lie above the threshold of 'normal' risk levels and they are those hazards which, given present or foreseeable technology, could reasonably be avoided. In the case of dentistry, for example, it is clear that the food industry contributes to a level of oral disease that rises well above a generous minimum level of disease that one would expect to be associated with a varied and interesting diet.

This is not to deny that vast improvements in food supply, diet and nutritional status have taken place since the industrial revolution. In fact, it is probably true to say that the advances in life expectancy in the industrial societies recorded since the nineteenth century probably owe more to advances in food supply and nutrition than they do to any other combination of factors (McKeown, 1976: 7). It is one of the ironies of the history of medicine that, just as certain long-term changes in diet have contributed substantially to improvements in life expectancy, so they have also had no small part in increasing our susceptibility to a range of chronic, degenerative disorders that are more characteristic of contemporary industrial society. In particular, increases in the intake of fat and sugar and decreasing amounts of dietary fibre are among some of the developments in our dietary patterns that have been held to account for the modern diseases of affluence.[3]

While many of these changes in dietary patterns can be attributed to commercial motives of profitability and the need to gain a competitive edge in the market, it cannot be denied that there is an all-important element of consumer choice and demand in these trends. It would be absurd to claim that such trends have been fostered and created by manipulative commercial interests and then foisted on an unwilling public. But the fact remains that even in the light of what we currently know about non-cariogenic substitutes (Scheinin *et al.,* 1974: 383; Newbrun and Frostell, 1978: 69-71), and given the enormous potential diversity of dietary life styles, the food industry has consistently fostered and developed dentally harmful patterns of food consumption. Without claiming too much for the power of advertising and the mass media, it is still highly plausible to suggest that the sweetening of baby foods (Shannon, 1978: 19-20) and the heavy promotion of cariogenic breakfast foods (Cornely, 1971: 10) — to mention just two marketing strategies aimed at the young — must have their effect in shaping the future direction of public demand. This is especially likely to be the case where, in contrast to the typical health education campaign, advertisers have merely to reinforce, rather than to counteract, attractive social values such as hedonism and personal self-indulgence. Apart from social barriers of this nature, there also remains the problem of an economic orthodoxy that dictates that effective prevention actually has a negative impact on measures of prosperity, while the production and marketing of cariogenic foods, and the repair of their ill-effects, contribute to economic growth according to standard criteria.[4]

To say that there are economic interests in the oral health field amounts to little more than saying that dentistry is an area of human concern and as such commands its share of human and material resources. But the significance of a 'medical-industrial complex' and the food and sugar lobbies is much more than this. To put it no more strongly, the interests of such economic blocs are dictated by commercial considerations that may or may not coincide with the broader public interest. In this instance, as in so many others, the case of medicine is the one that is more fully documented. What has been termed the 'medical-industrial complex' has become a crucial force in shaping the development of the medical system. While much is said about the importance of prevention, whole-person medicine, and community-based services, the tendency towards high-technology medicine, with its reliance on sophisticated surgical and pharmaceutical procedures, continues unchecked. If such trends in medical investment could be shown to contribute substantially to the improvement of the health of the community, there would be little cause for concern. The efficacy of many such developments is unproven, their impact on the health of the community very limited, and even negative in some instances, and their cost-effectiveness highly questionable.

In making just this point, McKinlay (1978) has drawn an illuminating parallel between health care manufacturing and the American motor vehicle industry. He argues that in the health field we can in principle identify medical procedures that are wholly, or in part, cost-effective; that is, techniques that have a definite beneficial effect on the individual's health status, and do this for a reasonable outlay of resources. In terms of McKinlay's parallel with the motor vehicle industry, what he is talking about here is the serviceable, utility vehicle that can perform a number of useful functions at a modest outlay: the 'Model T' of health care. But beyond this Model T level there is a great range of medical procedures and technologies that reflect almost entirely superfluous investment of resources, i.e. procedures which add nothing, or very little, to the effectiveness of health intervention. Like the gadgetry and gimmickry of the large American saloon, the sole aim of such investment is cosmetic and serves mainly to enhance the profit margins of the manufacturer. Just as the drive for profitability may encourage food manufacturers to promote harmful patterns of consumption, and just as similar motivations lie behind the opposition to adequate safety levels in the work environment and on the road, so it is that many medical procedures represent needless and excessive, and sometimes positively harmful, therapeutic developments. Furthermore, in some instances, firms with a responsibility for causing ill-health — say, tobacco companies — may also be involved in the medical supply industry. With the growing concentration and interconnectedness of modern industry, such linkages are likely to become increasingly common.

The crucial question, then, in what one might call the political economy of dentistry, is not so much whether there exist vested economic interests in the field — because clearly there do, and they constitute an essential economic infrastructure. Rather, the question is whether those interests that do exist contribute to unnecessary health risks or to pointlessly elaborate and sophisticated dental procedures. On the issue of health risks the case seems clear-cut. Even given what we presently know about sugar substitutes and about food alternatives, there is a clear case for those who would argue that we are needlessly 'manufacturing' caries. As far as the dental supply industry is concerned, the situation is a more subtle one and certainly less clear-cut. It becomes a matter of determining whether or not the resources channelled by the industry into elaborate equipment and expensive materials would be better used elsewhere.

One alternative avenue for resource allocation would be investment in fluoridation schemes. It could be argued that investment in elaborate dental technology has diverted resources from worthwhile prevention schemes like fluoridation. The cost-effectiveness of the fluoridation of public water supplies *vis à vis* other possible intervention strategies is beyond question (Backer Dirks *et al.,* 1978: 9-11; Meskin *et al.,* 1978: 304), though there is evidence that the fluoridation of salt may have similar effects and prove equally cost-effective (Marthaler *et al.,* 1978: 20). Yet, the population coverage of fluoridation is extremely limited. Could this be due — as has been argued in the case of health intervention — to the fact that elaborate treatment strategies are diverting resources away from adequate prevention? While this may be true in many respects — for example, the lack of social science research directed at understanding the many behavioural obstacles to prevention — the failure to achieve a wider coverage in the fluoridation of public water supplies reflects political problems in gaining its implementation, rather than any diversion of resources.

In fact, dentistry is rather different from medicine in this respect since it has nothing akin to the spectacular excesses of medical intervention. Furthermore, those extravagances that do exist — excessive crown and bridge work, elaborate orthodontics, 'full-mouth rehabilitations' (Howard, 1976: 12) — are attributable more to payment mechanisms and individual professional decisions rather than to the dental supply industry, a fact confirmed by the evidence of professional fraud and over-utilisation in the quality control studies of Medicaid in New York (Bellin and Kavaler, 1970). Of course, it may well be that profit-taking and excessive packaging and marketing cosmetics are adding substantially to the costs of dental care and, hence, to the financial burden on the community. But, in the absence of the sort of cost-benefit studies that have been carried out on some medical procedures, this 'cost-plus' factor remains the extent of the economic burden imposed on oral health care by the dental supply industry.

Aside from the effects of such economic interests as the food lobby and the dental supply industry there is the impact of organised dentistry itself. Within the broad confines of social structure and political tradition, the delivery system and its detailed functioning reflect a treatment philosophy, occupational ideology and a pattern of work organisation that is almost entirely of the dental profession's own making. This apparatus has been developed, of course, within the broad limitations imposed by a cultural tradition and by various economic, social and political interests. But the detailed impact of these factors is rather limited, if only because in dentistry — as in other skill- and knowledge- intensive areas of middle-class labour — the predominant form of occupational organisation is that of the profession which is able to provide considerable autonomy for the practitioner. Because of the complexity and esoteric nature of the work and because of certain protective features of work organisation — such as the loyalty of colleagues, social status, etc. — professionals enjoy an autonomy in their work that is unparalleled in other occupations. So, they are shielded to some extent from the influence of external factors and are able to dictate far more freely the routines and organisation of work.

Therefore, where economic, social or political influences may dictate certain broad tendencies in the oral health field — such as the level of oral disease, product and equipment range, social diversity of demand, the legal framework — it is the profession that interprets these tendencies and translates them into the daily routines of dentistry. It follows, then, that the extent to which the functioning of the dental system reflects any broader interests will depend significantly on the degree to which these broader interests coincide with those of the profession. Hence, the promotion of a new product or item of equipment is easier to achieve because it is much less likely to be viewed as a threat to the interests of the profession (in contrast to other measures likely to infringe the individual practitioner's freedom of movement, such as the correction of geographic maldistribution of resources, or quality control, or limitations on clinical autonomy (McKinlay, 1973: 80)).

Social Analysis and Policy Intervention

Modern diet and the food industry, the rise of the dental profession and the delivery system provide the main institutional features of contemporary dentistry. But what prospects are there for intervention and what lead can social analysis give us? An impression that may have been gained from much of the discussion and analysis that has preceded in earlier chapters is that the social context or environment of dentistry provides a complex, even chaotic, aspect; such is the apparent multiplicity of social factors affecting the organisation and delivery of care, and such the complex nature of the interaction of these factors, that it would be easy to interpret the situation as offering very little opportunity for deliberate and planned change. Certainly, it is difficult to exaggerate the complex and multi-faceted nature of the social environment in which dentistry has to function, and it would be a great disservice to the cause of the social sciences to suggest otherwise. Nevertheless, despite the evident complexity of the social context of dentistry, it *is* possible to identify a number of themes that underlie much of the discussion in previous chapters and that provide a more or less solid foundation for social analysis and policy intervention.

One major theme that emerges in any social analysis of dentistry is the distinction that is often drawn between the effects of cultural and non-cultural factors in conditioning the pattern of oral health in the community. Whether they be the analysis of oral care practice, dietary patterns, dental utilisation, treatment patterns or oral health status itself, the social factors highlighted in such analyses tend to fall into two quite distinct categories:

(1) the values, beliefs and attitudes that individuals learn and put into practice and that affect the way they care for their own health and use professional services; and
(2) the economic, material and physical factors that influence people's behaviour, the extent to which cultural items — like values and beliefs — are translated into practice, and condition the formation of such cultural traits in the first instance.

This broad division in the focus of social analysis applies equally to the activities of providers as it does to the behaviour of consumers; it runs through the discussion of etiology and the determination of oral health just as much as it affects the analysis of treatment, oral care and related patterns of behaviour. One area where the issue is perhaps most clearly articulated is that of dental utilisation; much of the debate in academic circles, and much policy discussion too, centres on whether attitudes, beliefs and values are the most important factors in affecting the way in which people use dental services, or whether non-cultural factors — such as physical and economic access — are more significant. Implicit in such very different emphases in analysis are quite contrasting strategies of policy intervention.

A second general theme that runs through much of the earlier discussion is the distinction that can be drawn between two broad levels of social analysis: that is, analysis at the level of the individual and of individual attributes such as beliefs, practices and personal economic resources, and analysis at the collective level of groups, organisations, institutions and cultural forms. The distinction is of course not quite as clearcut as this classification might imply; research and policy information, for example, is usually collected at an individual level, even though such information could well be used as a basis for collective strategies of intervention. Because so much health-related information is collected using social survey techniques, it is natural that much of the data that we have relates, in the first instance at least, to individual attributes like attitudes, behaviour and health status. However, the fact that such information is collected from individuals does not exclude its use in analyses at the group or collective level; individual data can quite simply be aggregated to give us information about collective phenomena such as dietary differences between countries, social group variations in health status and utilisation, etc.

Although it *is* possible to identify these two general themes underlying much of the discussion in previous chapters — the distinction between cultural and non-cultural factors, individual and collective levels of analysis — these two dimensions, or themes, of the discussion are rather closely intertwined and to separate them in the manner suggested might be considered artificial. In particular, it is clear that most accounts or explanations couched in terms of cultural factors tend also to stress the importance of individual attributes, rather than collective factors. Such a focus is implicit in the life-style concept and much work carried out in the tradition of health beliefs research. In other words, much of the discussion about the importance of values, beliefs and attitudes has been shifted from the rather abstract level of 'the lay health culture' to the far more concrete level of individual attitudes and behaviour. The natural policy developments that follow from such a shift in emphasis are those that focus on the modification of individual behaviour. Similarly, it would be easy to conclude from the earlier discussion that analyses presented in terms of economic, organisational and other non-cultural factors lead naturally to a more institutional or collective focus of interest, since much of the research carried out in this area has been concerned with issues involving the reform of the delivery system and changes in the profession itself.

Table 8.1: Social Analysis and Policy Intervention

Focus of Intervention	Focus of Analysis	
	Cultural	Non-Cultural
Collective	Content of mass media Training of providers Education of consumers	Delivery system 'Manufacturers of illness' The profession
Individual	Health education	Voluntary price 'signals' Private insurance

Although there *is* this natural alignment between type of analysis and form of intervention, there is actually no necessary connection between the two, as Table 8.1 shows. Although it would probably be true to say that most 'cultural' explanations tend to rely on methodologies and concepts in the tradition of life-style research and health beliefs, there is no essential reason why this should be so. Changes in institutional sources of information and attitude-formation could just as well be considered, though the barriers to implementation in this case are likely to be very much greater.[5] The case of material and non-cultural factors is similar. Implicit in the work of any investigators in this field is an agenda for major structural and institutional change. Yet, this does not preclude forms of intervention directed at individual providers and consumers.

Apart from these two dimensions – the focus of social analysis and the direction of policy intervention – a third theme that underlies much of the discussion in earlier chapters is the quite contrasting requirements of the two principal oral diseases, caries and periodontal disease; forms of analysis and strategies of intervention are found to vary quite markedly between these two conditions. More especially, given what we know about the etiology of these two disorders, the scope for more institutional forms of intervention seems greater in the case of caries than it is for periodontal disease. Because of the major importance of diet in the etiology of caries there is an opportunity for institutional intervention that does not exist in the case of periodontal disease where, by contrast, self-care seems to be more important.[6]

Table 8.2: Oral Condition and Policy Intervention

Stage of Intervention	Oral Condition	
	Caries	Periodontal Disease
Etiology	Diet Fluoridation	Oral care
Oral Care	Provider	Provider Consumer
Treatment	Limited preventive Major repair Prosthetics	Major preventive Limited repair Prosthetics

In Table 8.2 an attempt is made to compare some of the major differences in policy orientation that flow from the contrasting requirements of caries and periodontal disease. If we first consider the level of etiology, the options for intervention that are open to us are quite strikingly different for the two conditions. In the case of caries the options for intervention are both of an individual and an institutional nature; both diet and fluoridation can be approached either by directing resources at the individual or by carrying out certain institutional changes. To date, diet and fluoridation have been approached at quite different levels of intervention; while the emphasis for the former has been on changing individual dietary practices rather than on modifying the policies of the food industry,[7] fluoridation has generally been directed at the collective level — public water supplies — rather than at individual consumers.[8] In the case of periodontal disease, however, the opportunity for prevention seems to be almost entirely concentrated on the potential for individual preventive activity.

The issue of oral care provides the opportunity for strategies of institutional change for both conditions. Because provider services are important in both cases in maintaining oral health, the opportunity for collective intervention is equally available — both in the organisation and delivery of services and in dental education. Changes in both these areas would simultaneously improve access to care and lend a more preventive emphasis to professional practice. Economic sanctions — either directed on a voluntary basis at individual practitioners, or enforced on a collective basis — could reinforce preventive patterns of dental practice. The fact that in the case of periodontal disease there is also scope for self-care means that, again, the emphasis in this area is naturally on individual health actions.[9]

Treatment options for the two conditions are quite varied. While the great bulk of work carried out on the dentition is concerned with reconstruction and repair, the direction in which periodontal treatment has most scope for expansion is that of prevention and maintenance care. Because the problems of rationing and inequality become particularly acute in a treatment-oriented system, the only effective, long-term solutions in this area are those that by-pass the necessity for professional intervention on a regular basis. Such changes can only be effective if carried out at the institutional level. Hence, they are:

(1) changes in dental education that lay greater emphasis on the principles of maintenance care and prevention, rather than scattered inducements to individual practitioners;[10]

(2) radical initiatives in the deployment of auxiliary workers skilled in preventive work and able to increase the productivity of graduate dentists, rather than timid experimentation and meagre subsidies;[11]

(3) incentive systems that ration expensive (or extractive) treatment and that encourage maintenance care;[12]

(4) changes in the dental supply industry that foster the development of adequate technology and expertise for self-care and that reduce the incentive to elaborate, restorative care;

(5) strategies for prevention directed at the etiological stage.

Individual strategies are likely to be much less effective. They would involve health education programmes and schemes for selective and voluntary subsidisation of preventive dental practice.

Conclusion

There is little doubt that merely to alter the way in which dental care is financed is actually going to result in the intensification of the already heavy clinical emphasis of contemporary dentistry since, without the restraints of cost, the natural tendency would be to drive ever deeper into more elaborate and more active forms of clinical intervention. There will of course be some social benefits as well. The poor will be in a position to afford restorative care; orthodontic work will no longer be the prerogative of the middle class; crown and bridge work may increasingly substitute for early extraction and the fitting of dentures; the poor and the elderly will be able to afford more elaborate and more frequent prosthetic care. Each one of these developments amounts to a small, but significant, gain for various disadvantaged groups in society. But to be weighed against this: such gains will be achieved at massive cost; they will place enormous strain on the distributive system and introduce new, and more potent, inequalities — between different categories of patient and between different geographical areas; and they will barely make any impact at all on the overall oral health of the community.

If these problems are to be addressed, then, much more than just the payment system will require modification. The key to future change is probably the clinical model itself since it encapsulates so much of contemporary dentistry. Few substantial changes can take place in any other area of professional life — such as the service ethic, for example — without major modification of the clinical model itself, because it provides a theoretical justification and rationale for so much else that goes on in dentistry. Again, it is possible to argue that it is only the social sciences that can establish the basis for an alternative model of professional intervention.

The implications of such a change in emphasis are far-reaching. In the first place, it would mean abandoning, or at least greatly reducing, the sort of biochemical and other etiological work that is the mainstay of most scientific research in dentistry. Research of this kind contributes little to our understanding of the more global issues of oral health and, in fact, provides little more than a progressive refinement of detailed information on various disease processes within the confines of the mouth, disease processes about which we know a lot in any case. It is difficult to see what scientifically feasible discovery in this area would materially or substantially change any aspect of contemporary dental practice. By contrast, a shift in emphasis towards social science factors —

the social determination of diet, hazards at leisure and work, self-care, levels and styles of utilisation and treatment — would go far to completely reorientate dental practice in the direction of forms of intervention that would be less treatment-based and more preventive in emphasis.

Secondly, a social scientific perspective would do much to lay the basis for a realistic model of dental intervention. At present we are expected to accept the fiction that what goes on in dental practice can in large measure be traced to a specific body of theory and expertise applied to the everyday problems of oral health. The influence of economic incentive, clientele, the organisation of work, community context, commercial interest groups, colleague pressure, the availability of resources, and customary practice and tradition, all go entirely unacknowledged in such a fictional view of the world. These are all factors that materially affect the everyday routine of dental practice and that could be shaped and modified in such a way as to improve the quality and distribution of dental care.

Finally, in identifying the impact of non-clinical factors and in subjecting established professional beliefs and practices to scrutiny, the social sciences may encourage a far more self-conscious and flexible approach to what are otherwise rather uncritically accepted nostrums of dental belief and practice. Of course, taken to its extreme, such a searching scrutiny would merely substitute an aimless relativism for the (rather specious) precision and certainty of the clinical model. But developed in an intelligent and flexible manner, the self-analysis and critical scrutiny encouraged by the social sciences would do much to broaden the scope of dentistry and, in effect, foster its emergence as a true science of oral health rather than the craft of dental treatment it is otherwise destined to remain.

Notes

1. To some extent the same problem applies in social definitions of illness. Parsons' emphasis on the attribution of sickness by a medical practitioner as being the feature distinguishing illness from other forms of deviance, such as crime, does not provide a ready basis for the analysis of the social etiology of illness (Twaddle, 1973: 756).

2. Parsons' formulation of health and illness in terms of the capacity to perform institutionalised social roles at least has the merit of focusing attention on the broader social consequences of different health conditions, as against the strictly social-psychological interpretations of medical practice (Kasl, 1974: 434). Death and disease in the workplace provide grounds for concern from the point of

view of the costs to society for production lost due to ill-health. They also provide a clear etiological focus since many conditions can be traced to aspects of the work environment (A. Miller, 1975: 1218-19).

3. The major changes in diet have been in the direction of more atherogenic foods (saturated fats, cholesterol), more sugar and less whole grain products. Nearly 50 per cent of all deaths are attributable to atherosclerotic processes (Winikoff, 1977: 552). The decrease in the intake of dietary fibre and the associated increase in the consumption of fat has been linked to the changing pattern of heart disease, although anomalous research findings have also been reported (Krilshevsky, 1976: 626). Items of modern diet, such as fat intake and dietary fibre, have also been linked to cancer (Alcantara and Speckman, 1976).

4. For a critique of orthodox criteria of economic performance such as GNP, see Draper *et al.* (1976: 24).

5. An interesting example of the diffusion of preventive health practices in a population is given by Ellenbogen *et al.* (1968). Education and age were the most important factors governing acceptance of the preventive practices, one of which was dental service use.

6. Periodontal disease may not be entirely unrelated to diet. Goldberg (1977: 154) claims that nutrition may affect the rate and severity of periodontal disease, even while it may not be important in initiating the disease.

7. Norway is attempting to introduce a national nutrition policy which, instead of focusing on individual behaviour, is intended to change the pattern of food production and distribution (Ringen, 1979).

8. The extent of fluoridation is, however, still rather limited. Of 31 countries recently reviewed in Europe by WHO, only three had more than 10 per cent of the population served by fluoridated water supplies. Five countries had more than 10 per cent of school children on topical fluoride application (Kostlan, 1972).

9. For a critique of the self-care concept, see Kronenfeld (1979).

10. Maxwell (1974: 44) claims that the economics of current payment mechanisms in dentistry are such as to discourage regular check-ups and early treatment.

11. The WHO study of dental manpower systems found that 60-70 per cent of dentists interviewed in the five countries saw a need for the increased use of dental auxiliaries (Bonito and Cohen, 1978). It would appear, then, that the profession is at least open to the idea. In Saskatchewan, the introduction of school dental nurses was found to have no ill-effects on the incomes of the private dental practitioners (Lewis, 1978), suggesting that experimentation with dental auxiliaries can go quite far without threatening the interests of the dental profession.

12. Knutson (1979) claims that many questionable procedures would have to be excluded from any comprehensive third-party coverage of costs. These would include: fixed bridges for the back of the mouth; major periodontal surgery; much orthodontic work in the 6-12 age group; and probably treatment of the primary (or deciduous) teeth.

BIBLIOGRAPHY

Abramovitz, J. and Berg, L.E. 'A Four-Year Study of the Utilization of
    Dental Assistants with Expanded Functions', *Journal of the American
    Dental Association,* 87 (1973)
Adams, K. and Fraser, R.D. 'Introduction and Overview' in R.D. Fraser
    (ed.), *Symposium on Health Care Economics* (Industrial Relations
    Centre, Kingston, 1976)
Addy, M. and Edmunds, S. 'Effectiveness of Methods of Teaching Dental
    Health to 9-10 Year Old Schoolchildren in the United Kingdom',
    Community Dentistry and Oral Epidemiology, 5 (1977)
Agerback, N. *et al.* 'Effect of Professional Toothcleaning Every Third
    Week on Gingivitis and Dental Caries in Children', *Community
    Dentistry and Oral Epidemiology,* 6 (1977)
Agerberg, G. and Carlsson, G.E. 'Functional Disorders of the Masticatory
    System. I. Distribution of Symptoms According to Age and Sex as
    Judged from Investigation by Questionnaire', *Acta Odontologica
    Scandinavica,* 30 (1972)
—— 'Functional Disorders of the Masticatory System. II. Symptoms in
    Relation to Impaired Motility of the Mandible as Judged from
    Investigation by Questionnaire', *Acta Odontologica Scandinavica,* 31
    (1973)
Ainamo, J. 'Awareness of the Presence of Dental Caries and Gingival
    Inflammation in Young Adult Males', *Acta Odontologica Scandinavica,*
    30 (1972)
Ainamo, J. and Holmberg, S. 'A Retrospective Longitudinal Study of
    Caries Prevalence During and 7 Years After Free Dental Care at
    School in Finland', *Community Dentistry and Oral Epidemiology,* 1
    (1973)
Akers, L. and Quinney, R. 'Differential Organization of Health
    Professions: A Comparative Analysis', *American Sociological Review,*
    33 (1968)
Alcantara, E.N. and Speckman, L.S. 'Diet, Nutrition and Cancer',
    Americal Journal of Clinical Nutrition, 29 (1976)
Allman, H.B. 'Man is Not a Giant Rat', *Journal of Public Health
    Dentistry,* 31 (1971)
Allred, H. *The Training and Use of Dental Auxiliary Personnel* (WHO
    Regional Office for Europe, Copenhagen, 1977)

Anaise, J.Z. 'Prevalence of Dental Caries among Workers in the Sweets Industry in Israel', *Community Dentistry and Oral Epidemiology,* 6 (1978)

Andersen, R. and Newman, J.F. 'Societal and Individual Determinants of Medical Care Utilization in the United States', *Milbank Memorial Fund Quarterly,* 51 (1973)

Andersen, R. *et al.* (eds.) *Equity in Health Services: Empirical Analyses in Social Policy* (Ballinger, Cambridge Mass., 1975)

— *Two Decades of Health Services: Social Survey Trends in Use and Expenditure* (Ballinger, Cambridge Mass., 1976)

Anderson, O.W. 'Styles of Planning Health Services: The United States, Sweden, and England', *International Journal of Health Services,* 1 (1971)

— 'The Politics of Universal Health Insurance in the United States: An Interpretation', *International Journal of Health Services,* 2 (1972)

Anderson, R.J. *et al.* 'Dental Caries Experience and Treatment Patterns. Social Differences in 1,252 University Students', *British Dental Journal,* 131 (1971)

Antoft, P.E. *et al.* 'Social Inequality and Caries Studies in 1,719 Danish Military Recruits', *Community Dentistry and Oral Epidemiology,* 2 (1974)

Antonovsky, A. and Kats, R. 'The Model Dental Patient: An Empirical Study of Preventive Health Behavior', *Social Science and Medicine,* 4 (1970)

Armstrong, D. 'The Decline of the Medical Hegemony: A Review of Government Reports During the NHS', *Social Science and Medicine,* 10 (1976)

— 'Clinical Sense and Clinical Science', *Social Science and Medicine,* 11 (1977)

— 'The Emancipation of Biographical Medicine', *Social Science and Medicine,* 13A (1979)

Asgis, A.J. 'The Rise and Growth of the Stomatologic Movement in America', *Journal of Dental Research,* 11 (1931)

Avery, K.T. 'The Oral Health Status of Migrant and Seasonal Farm-workers and Their Families in Florida', *Community Dentistry and Epidemiology,* 4 (1976)

Axelsson, P. *et al.* 'The Effect of Various Plaque Control Measures on Gingivitis and Caries in Schoolchildren', *Community Dentistry and Oral Epidemiology,* 4 (1976)

Backer Dirks, O. *et al.* 'Caries — Preventive Water Fluoridation', *Caries Research,* 12 (Suppl. 1) (1978)

Bagramian, R.A. and Russell, A.L. 'Epidemiologic Study of Dental Caries Experience and Between-Meal Eating Patterns', *Journal of Dental Research,* 52 (1973)

Bagramian, R.A. *et al.* 'Diet Patterns and Dental Caries in Third Grade United States Children', *Community Dentistry and Oral Epidemiology,* 2 (1974)

Bailit, H.L. 'Effectiveness of Personal Dental Services on Improving Oral Health', *Journal of Public Health Dentistry,* 38 (1978)

Bailit, H.L. *et al.* 'Controlling the Cost of Dental Care', *American Journal of Public Health,* 69 (1979)

Barenthin, I. 'A Review and Discussion of Goals in Community Dentistry', *Community Dentistry and Oral Epidemiology,* 3 (1975)

—— 'Dental Insurance and Equity of Access to Dental Services', *Community Dentistry and Oral Epidemiology,* 4 (1976)

—— 'Dental Health Status and Dental Satisfaction', *International Journal of Epidemiology,* 6 (1977)

Baric, L. 'Recognition of the "At-Risk" Role: A Means to Influence Health Behavior', *International Journal of Health Education,* 12 (1969)

Beal, J.F. and Dowell, T.B. 'Edentulousness and Attendance Patterns in England and Wales, 1968-1977', *British Dental Journal,* 143 (1977)

Becker, M.H. 'The Health Belief Model and Sick Role Behavior', *Health Education Monograph,* 2 (1974)

Becker, M.H. and Maiman, L. 'Sociobehavioral Determinants of Compliance with Health and Medical Care Recommendations', *Medical Care,* 13 (1975)

Becker, M.H. *et al.* 'Predicting Mother's Compliance with Pediatric Medical Regimens', *Journal of Pediatrics,* 81 (1972)

—— 'The Health Belief Model and Prediction of Dietary Compliance: A Field Experiment', *Journal of Health and Social Behavior,* 18 (1977a)

—— 'Selected Psychosocial Models and Correlates of Individual Health-Related Behaviors', *Medical Care,* 15 (1977b)

Bell, D. *The End of Ideology; On the Exhaustion of Political Ideas in the Fifties,* 2nd edn. (Free Press, New York, 1965)

—— *The Coming of Post-Industrial Society; A Venture in Social Forecasting* (Basic Books, New York, 1973)

Bellin, L.E. and Kavaler, F. 'Policing Publicly Funded Health Care for Poor Quality, Over-Utilization, and Fraud — The New York City Medicaid Experience', *American Journal of Public Health,* 60 (1970)

Belloc, N.B. 'Relationship of Health Practices and Mortality', *Preventive Medicine,* 2 (1973)

Belloc, N.B. and Breslow, L. 'Relationship Between Physical Health Status and Health Practices', *Preventive Medicine,* 1 (1972)

Bennie, A.M. *et al.* 'Five Years of Community Preventive Dentistry and Health Education in the County of Sutherland, Scotland', *Community Dentistry and Oral Epidemiology,* 6 (1976)

Berenie, J.T. *et al.* 'The Effect of Toothbrushing Frequency on Oral Hygiene and Gingival Health in Schoolchildren: A Reassessment After 2½ Years', *Journal of Public Health Dentistry,* 36 (1976)

Berkanovic, E. 'Lay Conceptions of the Sick Role', *Social Forces,* 51 (1972)

Berlant, J.L. *Profession and Monopoly: A Study of Medicine in the United States and Great Britain* (University of California Press, London, 1975)

Berliner, H.S. 'A Larger Perspective on the Flexner Report', *International Journal of Health Services,* 5 (1975)

Bibby, B. 'Do We Tell the Truth About Preventing Caries?', *Journal of Dentistry of Children,* 33 (1966)

—— 'The Cariogenicity of Snack Foods and Confections', *Journal of the American Dental Association,* 90 (1975)

Bice, T.W. *et al.* 'Socioeconomic Status and Use of Physician Services: A Reconsideration', *Medical Care,* 10 (1972)

Blaugh, L.E. 'Relation Between Dental and Medical Education', *Journal of the American Dental Association,* 22 (1935)

Blaxter, M. 'Social Class and Health Inequalities' in C.O. Carter and J. Peel (eds.), *Equalities and Inequalities in Health* (Academic Press, London, 1976)

Bloom, S.W. 'The Sociology of Medical Education', *Milbank Memorial Fund Quarterly,* 43 (1965)

Bloom, S.W. and Wilson, R.N. 'Patient-Practitioner Relationships' in H.E. Freeman *et al.* (eds.), *Handbook of Medical Sociology* 2nd edn. (Prentice-Hall, Englewood Cliffs, N.J., 1972)

Boggs, D.G. and Schwartz, M.A. 'Determination of Optimal Time Lapses for Recall of Patients in an Incremental Dental Care Program', *Journal of the American Dental Association,* 90 (1975)

Bonito, A.J. and Cohen, L.K. 'Characteristics of Dental Providers and Practices in Australia, Federal Republic of Germany, Japan, New Zealand, Norway and the U.S.' (Unpublished Paper Presented to 66th. FDI Congress, Madrid, 1978)

Boudreau, T.J. and Rivard, J.-Y. 'An Evaluation of Different Methods for Remunerating Physicians' in R.D. Fraser (ed.), *Symposium on Health Care Economics* (Industrial Relations Centre, Kingston, 1976)

Bowler, M.K. *et al.* 'The Political Economy of National Health Insurance: Policy Analysis and Policy Evaluation', *Journal of Health Politics, Policy and Law,* 2 (1977)

Breslow, L. 'A Quantitative Approach to the WHO Definition of Health: Physical, Mental and Social Well-Being', *International Journal of Epidemiology,* 1 (1972)

Bridgstock, M. 'Professions and Social Background: The Work Organisation of General Practitioners', *Sociological Review,* 24 (1976)

British Dental Association, 'Economies of Scale in Dental Practice', *British Dental Journal,* 141 (1976)

Bureau of Economic Research and Statistics, 'A Motivational Study of Dental Care', *Journal of the American Dental Association,* 56 (1958)

Burkitt, D.P. 'Diseases of Modern Economic Development' in G.M. Howe and J.A. Loraine (eds.), *Environmental Medicine* (Heinemann, London, 1973)

Burman, R. 'The Dentition of Children in the Island of Lewis', *British Dental Journal,* 116 (1964)

Burt, B.A. 'The Administration of Public Dental Treatment Programmes' in G.L. Slack and B.A. Burt (eds.), *Dental Public Health: An Introduction to Community Dentistry* (John Wright and Sons, Bristol, 1974)

—— 'Influences for Change in the Dental Health Status of Populations: An Historical Perspective', *Journal of Public Health Dentistry,* 38 (1978)

Carr-Saunders, A.M. and Wilson, P.A. *The Professions* (Frank Cass, London, 1933)

Cartwright, A. *et al. Life Before Death* (Routledge and Kegan Paul, London, 1973)

Castells, M. 'The Service Economy and Postindustrial Society: A Sociological Critique', *International Journal of Health Services,* 6 (1976)

Castles, F.G. and McKinlay, R.D. 'Public Welfare Provision, Scandinavia, and the Sheer Futility of the Sociological Approach to Politics', *British Journal of Political Science,* 9 (1979)

Chubin, D.E. and Studer, K.E. 'The Politics of Cancer', *Theory and Society,* 6 (1978)

Clancy, K.L. *et al.* 'Snack Food Intake of Adolescents and Caries Development', *Journal of Dental Research,* 56 (1977)

—— 'Snack Food Consumption of 12 Year Old Inner-City Children and Its Relationship to Oral Health', *Journal of Public Health Dentistry,* 38 (1978)

Cleaton-Jones, P. *et al.* 'Dental Caries in Rural and Urban Black Preschoolchildren', *Community Dentistry and Oral Epidemiology,* 6 (1978)

Cochrane, A.L. *Effectiveness and Efficiency: Random Reflections on the Health Service* (Nuffield Provincial Hospitals Trust, London, 1972)

Cohen, L.K. 'Social Psychological Factors Associated with Malocclusion', *International Dental Journal,* 20 (1970)

Cohen, L.K. and Fusillo, A.E. 'Public Concern About Provision of Dental Care', *Journal of Public Health Dentistry,* 31 (1971)

Cohen, L.K. and Jago, J.D. 'Toward the Formulation of Sociodental Indicators', *International Journal of Health Services,* 6 (1976)

Cohen, L.K. *et al.* 'Toothbrushing: Public Opinion and Dental Research', *Journal of Oral Therapeutics and Pharmacology,* 4 (1967)

Cole, R.B. and Cohen, L.K. 'Dental Manpower: Estimating Resources and Requirements', *Milbank Memorial Fund Quarterly,* 49 (1971)

Coleman, J.S. *et al. Medical Innovation* (Bobbs Merrill, Indianapolis, 1966)

Colombotos, J. *et al.* 'Physicians View National Health Insurance: A National Study', *Medical Care,* 13 (1975)

Comaroff, J. 'A Bitter Pill to Swallow: Placebo Therapy in General Practice', *Sociological Review,* 24 (1976a)

—— 'Communicating Information About Non-Fatal Illness: The Strategies of a Group of General Practitioners', *Sociological Review,* 24 (1976b)

—— 'Medicine and Culture: Some Anthropological Perspectives', *Social Science and Medicine,* 12B (1978)

Cook, P.J. and Walker, R.O. 'The Geographical Distribution of Dental Care in the United Kingdom', *British Dental Journal,* 122 (1967)

Cooper, J.A. 'USSR and US Health Policies', *New England Journal of Medicine,* 286 (1972)

Cooper, M. *Rationing Health Care* (Croom Helm, London, 1975)

Cordtz, D. 'Change Begins in the Doctor's Office', *Fortune,* 81 (1970)

Cornely, P.B. 'The Hidden Enemies of Health and the American Public Health Association', *American Journal of Public Health,* 61 (1971)

Craft, M. and Sheiham, A. 'Attitudes to Prevention Amongst Dental Practitioners: A Comparison Between the North and South of England', *British Dental Journal,* 141 (1976)

Cussler, M. and Gordon, E.W. *Dentists, Patients, and Auxiliaries* (University of Pittsburgh Press, Pittsburgh, 1968)

Davis, A. and Horobin, G. 'Conclusion — Problems of Patienthood' in A. Davis and G. Horobin (eds.), *Medical Encounters: The Experience of Illness and Treatment* (Croom Helm, London, 1977)

Dennison, D. 'Social Class Variables Related to Health Instruction', *American Journal of Public Health,* 62 (1972)

DHSS, *Prevention and Health: Everybody's Business* (HMSO, London, 1976)

De Stefano, T.M. 'Stomatology Revisited: The Solution for Professional Dentistry in American Society', *Journal of the American College of Dentists,* 42 (1975)

Dodd, D.M. 'The Emergence of Local Authority Dentistry from the Complex of a Developing Public Health System', *Public Health (London),* 82 (1968)

Doherty, N. 'Social and Delivery Factors in the Cost of Dental Care', *Medical Care,* 16 (1978)

Doherty, N. and Horowitz, P. 'Normal Returns and Profits to Private Dentists', *Journal of Dental Research,* 58 (Special Issue A) (1979)

Doherty, N. and Vivian, S.L. 'Costs of Publicly Financed Dental Care for Children in Three Different Types of Practice Settings', *Journal of Public Health Dentistry,* 36 (1976)

Donnison, J.M. 'The Battle for Midwife Registration – A Case-Study in Medical and Feminist Politics', *Social History of Medicine Bulletin,* 14 (1974)

Douglas, B.L. 'The "Free-Choice" and "Doctor-Patient" Myths', *New York State Dental Journal,* 37 (1971)

Draker, H.L. 'Judgments of Peers in Assessing the Orthodontic Handicap', *Journal of Public Health Dentistry,* 30 (1970)

Draper, P. *et al. Health, Money and the NHS* (Unit for the Study of Health Policy, London, 1976)

Dressel, H.W. 'A Brief History of Dental Corporations in the USA', *Journal of the Maryland State Dental Association,* 12 (1969)

Duany, L.F. *et al.* 'Epidemiologic Studies of Caries-Free and Caries-Active Students', *Journal of Dental Research,* 51 (1972)

Dudding, N.J. *et al.* 'Patient Reactions to Brushing Teeth with Water, Dentifrice or Salt and Soda', *Journal of Periodontology,* 31 (1960)

Dunlop, D.W. 'Alternatives to "Modern" Health Delivery Systems in Africa: Public Policy Issues', *Social Science and Medicine,* 9 (1975)

Dunning, J.M. *Principles of Dental Public Health,* 2nd edn. (Harvard University Press, Cambridge Mass., 1970)

Easlick, K.A. (ed.), 'An Evaluation of the Effect of Dental Foci of Infection on Health', *Journal of the American Dental Association,* 42 (1951)

Eaton, G. and Webb, B. 'Boundary Encroachment: Pharmacists in the Clinical Setting', *Sociology of Health and Illness,* 1 (1979)

Editorial, 'Dental Hygienists', *British Dental Journal,* 137 (1974)

Elderton, R.J. 'The Causes of Failure of Restorations: Literature Review of Clinical Investigations', *Journal of Dentistry,* 4 (1976a)

— 'The Prevalance of Failure of Restorations: A Literature Review', *Journal of Dentistry,* 4 (1976b)

Ellenbogen, B.L. *et al.* 'The Diffusion of Two Preventive Health Practices', *Inquiry,* 5 (1968)

Elliott, P. *The Sociology of the Professions* (Macmillan, London, 1972)

— 'Professional Ideology and Social Situation', *Sociological Review,* 21 (1973)

Ennis, J. *The Story of the Federation Dentaire Internationale, 1900-1962* (FDI, London, 1967)

Ettinger, R.L. 'An Evaluation of the Attitudes of a Group of Elderly Edentulous Patients to Dentists, Dentures, and Dentistry', *The Dental Practitioner and Dental Record,* 22 (1971)

— 'Diet, Nutrition and Masticatory Ability in a Group of Elderly Edentulous Patients', *Australian Dental Journal,* 18 (1973)

Faltermeyer, E.K. 'Better Care at Less Cost Without Miracles', *Fortune,* 81 (1970)

Fanshel, S. 'A Meaningful Measure of Health for Epidemiology', *International Journal of Epidemiology,* 1 (1972)

Feldstein, P.J. *Health Associations and the Demand for Legislation: The Political Economy of Health* (Ballinger, Cambridge Mass., 1977)

Fereday, R.C. 'Social Dentistry and Private Practice in the Federal Republic of Germany', *British Dental Journal,* 128 (1970)

Field, M.G. 'American and Soviet Medical Manpower: Growth and Evolution, 1910-1970', *International Journal of Health Services,* 5 (1975)

Foucault, M. *Birth of the Clinic* (Tavistock, London, 1973)

Fox, R.C. 'The Medicalization and Remedicalization of American Society' in J. Knowles (ed.), *Doing Better and Feeling Worse: Health in the U.S.* (W.W. Norton, New York, 1977)

Frankenberg, R. 'Functionalism and After? Theory and Developments in Social Science Applied to the Health Field', *International Journal of Health Services,* 4 (1974)

Franks, A.S.T. 'The Social Character of Temperomandibular Joint Dysfunction', *The Dental Practitioner and Dental Record,* 15 (1964)

Frazier, P.J. 'A New Look at Dental Health Education in Community Programmes', *Dental Hygiene,* 52 (1978)

Freidson, E. 'Client Control and Medical Practice', *American Journal of Sociology,* 65 (1960)

—— 'Review Essay: Health Factories, the New Industrial Sociology',
    Social Problems, 14 (1966-7)
—— *Professional Dominance* (Atherton Press, New York, 1970)
—— 'The Organization of Medical Practice' in H.E. Freeman *et al.* (eds.),
    Handbook of Medical Sociology, 2nd. edn. (Prentice-Hall, Englewood
    Cliffs, N.J., 1972)
—— 'Prepaid Group Practice and the New "Demanding Patient"', *Milbank
    Memorial Fund Quarterly (Health and Society),* 51 (1973a)
—— 'Professionalization and the Organization of Middle-Class Labour in
    Postindustrial Society' in P. Halmos (ed.), *Professionalisation and
    Social Change* (Sociological Review Monograph, University of Keele,
    1973b)
Freidson, E. and Feldman, J.J. 'The Public Looks at Dental Care',
    Journal of the American Dental Association, 57 (1958)
Freihofer, H. 'The Image of Dentistry: Continental Europe',
    International Dental Journal, 14 (1964)
Freymann, J.G. 'Medicine's Great Schism: Prevention Vs. Cure. An
    Historical Interpretation', *Medical Care,* 13 (1975)
Friedman, J.W. 'The Orthodontic Handicap; A Critique', *Journal of
    Public Health Dentistry,* 31 (1971)
Frostell, G. and Ericsson, Y. 'Anti-Plaque Therapeutics in Caries
    Prevention', *Caries Research,* 12 (Suppl. 1) (1978)
Fuchs, V. 'Health Care and the United States Economic System',
    Milbank Memorial Fund Quarterly (Health and Society), 50 (1972)
Galanter, R.B. 'To the Victim Belong the Flaws', *American Journal of
    Public Health,* 67 (1977)
Garcia, J. and Juarez, R.Z. 'Utilization of Dental Health Services by
    Chicanos and Anglos', *Journal of Health and Social Behavior,* 19 (1978)
Geertsen, R. *et al.* 'A Re-Examination of Suchman's Views on Social
    Factors in Health Care Utilization', *Journal of Health and Social
    Behavior,* 16 (1975)
Geertson, H.R. and Gray, R.M. 'Familistic Orientation and Inclination
    Toward Adopting the Sick Role', *Journal of Marriage and the Family,*
    32 (1970)
Gerson, L.W. 'Expectations of "Sick Role" Exemptions for Dental
    Problems', *Journal of the Canadian Dental Association,* 38 (1972)
Giddon, D.B. 'The Mouth and the Quality of Life', *New York Journal of
    Dentistry,* 48 (1978)
Gies, W.J. *Dental Education in the United States and Canada: A Report
    to the Carnegie Foundation for the Advancement of Teaching*
    (Carnegie, New York, 1926)

Gill, D.G. 'The British NHS: Professional Determinants of Administrative Structure', *International Journal of Health Services*, 1 (1971)

Glass, R.L. and Fleisch, S. 'Diet and Dental Caries: Dental Caries Incidence and the Consumption of Ready-to-Eat Cereals', *Journal of the American Dental Association*, 88 (1974)

Glass, R.L. *et al.* 'Secular Trends in the Prevalence of Caries', *Journal of Public Health Dentistry*, 33 (1973)

Goldberg, H.J.V. 'Interaction of Nutritional Factors in Oral Hygiene and Oral Health' in H.J.V. Goldberg and L.W. Ripa (eds.), *Oral Hygiene and Oral Health* (Charles C. Thomas, Springfield Ill., 1977)

Goldberg, H.J.V. and Hagin, H.A. 'Socialized Dentistry in Great Britain: An Historical Perspective', *Bulletin of the History of Dentistry*, 23 (1975)

Goldman, L. 'Factors Related to Physicians' Medical and Political Attitudes: A Documentation of Intraprofessional Variations', *Journal of Health and Social Behavior*, 15 (1974)

Goldstein, M.S. 'Physical Status of Men Examined Through Selective Service in World War II', *Public Health Reports*, 66 (1951)

Goose, D.H. and Gittus, E. 'Infant Feeding Methods and Dental Caries', *Public Health*, 82 (1968)

Gove, W.R. 'Sex Differences in Mental Illness Among Adult Men and Women: An Evaluation of Four Questions Raised Regarding the Evidence on the Higher Rates of Women', *Social Science and Medicine*, 12B (1978)

Gove, W.R. and Herb, T. 'Stress and Mental Illness Among the Young: A Comparison of the Sexes', *Social Forces*, 53 (1974)

Graves, R.C. *et al.*, 'A Comparison of the Effectiveness of the "Tooth-keeper" and a Traditional Dental Health Education Program', *Journal of Public Health Dentistry*, 35 (1975)

Grewe, J.M. and Hagan, D.V. 'Malocclusion Indices: A Comparative Evaluation', *American Journal of Orthodontics*, 61 (1972)

Groot, L.M.J. 'Postindustrial Europe and Its Health Care: Views of an Insider', *International Journal of Health Services*, 2 (1972)

Gullett, D.W. *A History of Dentistry in Canada* (University of Toronto Press, Toronto, 1971)

Gustafsson, B.E. *et al.* 'The Vipeholm Dental Caries Study. The Effect of Different Levels of Carbohydrate Intake on Caries Activity in 436 Individuals Observed for 5 Years', *Acta Odontologica Scandinavica*, 11 (1954)

Gyarmati, K.G. 'The Doctrine of the Professions', *International Social*

Science Journal, 27 (1975)

Haefner, D.P. 'The Health Belief Model and Preventive Dental Behavior', *Health Education Monograph,* 2 (1974)

Haefner, D.P. *et al.* 'Preventive Action in Dental Disease; Tuberculosis and Cancer', *Public Health Reports,* 82 (1967)

Hall, O. 'The Stages of a Medical Career', *American Journal of Sociology,* 53 (1948)

— 'Types of Medical Career', *American Journal of Sociology,* 55 (1949)

Halmos, P. *The Personal Service Society* (Constable, London 1969)

Hamilton, A.I. 'An Economic Analysis of Dental Practice', *Journal of the American Dental Association,* 66 (1963)

Hamilton, B. 'The Medical Professions in the Eighteenth Century', *Economic History Review,* 4 (1951)

Hamp, S.-E. *et al.* 'Effect of a Field Program Based on Systematic Plaque Control on Caries and Gingivitis in Schoolchildren After 3 Years', *Community Dentistry and Oral Epidemiology,* 6 (1978)

Hankin, J. *et al.* 'Genetic and Epidemiologic Studies of Oral Characteristics in Hawaii's Schoolchildren: Dietary Patterns and Caries Prevalence', *Journal of Dental Research,* 52 (1973)

Hankin, R.A. 'The Cost of Providing Restorative Dentistry in an Alternative Delivery Mode', *Journal of Public Health Dentistry,* 37 (1977)

Hardwick, J.L. 'The Incidence and Distribution of Caries Throughout the Ages in Relation to the Englishman's Diet', *British Dental Journal,* 108 (1960)

Hargreaves, J.A. 'Changes in Diet and Dental Health of Children Living in the Scottish Island of Lewis', *Caries Research,* 6 (1972)

Harrington, C. 'Medical Ideologies in Conflict', *Medical Care,* 13 (1975)

Heifetz, S.B. *et al.* 'Prevalence of Dental Caries in White and Black Children in Nelson County, Virginia, a Rural Southern Community', *Journal of Public Health Dentistry,* 36 (1976)

Hellman, S. 'The Dentist and Preventive Dental Health Information', *Health Education Monograph,* 4 (1976)

Helöe, B. and Helöe, L.A. 'Characteristics of a Group of Patients with Temporormandibular Joint Disorders', *Community Dentistry and Oral Epidemiology,* 3 (1975)

Helöe, L.A. and König, K.G. 'Oral Hygiene and Educational Programs for Caries Prevention', *Caries Research,* 12 (Suppl. 1) (1978)

Hemminki, E. and Pesonen, T. 'An Inquiry into Associations Between Leading Physicians and the Drug Industry in Finland', *Social Science and Medicine,* 11 (1977)

Hewat, R.E.T. and Eastcott, D.F. *Dental Caries in New Zealand* (Medical Research Council, Christchurch (New Zealand), 1956)

Holloway, P. 'The Success of Restorative Dentistry?', *International Dental Journal,* 25 (1975)

Holloway, P. *et al.* 'Dental Disease in Tristan da Cunha', *British Dental Journal,* 115 (1963)

Holloway, S. 'Medical Education in England, 1830-1858: A Sociological Analysis', *History,* 49 (1964)

— 'The Apothecaries Act, 1815: A Reinterpretation', *Medical History,* 10 (1966)

Holm, A.-K. 'A Longitudinal Study of Dental Health in Swedish Children Aged 3-5 Years', *Community Dentistry and Oral Epidemiology,* 3 (1975)

Holm A.-K. *et al.* 'A Comparative Study of Oral Health as Related to General Health, Food Habits and Socioeconomic Conditions of 4-Year Old Swedish Children', *Community Dentistry and Oral Epidemiology,* 3 (1975)

Horowitz, A.M. *et al.* 'Effects of Supervised Daily Dental Plaque Removal by Children: II. 24 Months' Results', *Journal of Public Health Dentistry,* 37 (1977)

Howard, C. 'Personal Preventive Procedures', *Proceedings, 83rd Congress, Royal Society of Health,* 1976

Iglehart, J.K. 'The Carter Administration's Health Budget: Charting New Priorities with Limited Dollars', *Milbank Memorial Fund Quarterly (Health and Society),* 56 (1978)

Illich, I. 'Disabling Professions' in I. Illich *et al.* (eds.), *Disabling Professions* (Marion Boyars, London, 1977)

Infante, P.F. and Owen, G.M. 'Dental Caries and Levels of Treatment for School Children by Geographical Region, Socioeconomic Status, Race, and Size of Community', *Journal of Public Health Dentistry,* 35 (1975)

Infante, P.F. and Russell, A.L. 'An Epidemiologic Study of Dental Caries in Preschool Children in the United States by Race and Socioeconomic Level', *Journal of Dental Research,* 53 (1974)

Ingervall, B. *et al.* 'Prevalence and Awareness of Malocclusion in Swedish Men', *Community Dentistry and Oral Epidemiology,* 6 (1978)

IADR, '57th General Session, IADR', *Journal of Dental Research,* 58 (Special Issue A) (1979)

Ivashchenko, G.M. 'The History of Stomatology in the USSR', *International Dental Journal,* 19 (1970)

Jaccard, J.A. 'Theoretical Analysis of Selected Factors Important to

Health Education Strategies', *Health Education Monograph,* 3 (1975)

Jackson, D. 'An Epidemiological Study of Dental Caries Prevalence in Adults', *Archives of Oral Biology,* 6 (1961)

—— 'Measuring Restorative Dental Care in Communities', *British Dental Journal,* 134 (1973)

—— 'Caries Experience in English Children and Young Adults During the Years 1947-1972', *British Dental Journal,* 137 (1974)

Jago, J.D. 'The Epidemiology of Dental Occlusion; A Critical Appraisal', *Journal of Public Health Dentistry,* 34 (1974)

James, P.M.C. and Beal, J.F. 'Dental Epidemiology and Survey Procedures' in G.L. Slack and B.A. Burt (eds.), *Dental Public Health: An Introduction to Community Dentistry* (John Wright and Sons, Bristol, 1974)

Jeffery, R. 'Allopathic Medicine in India: A Case of Deprofessionalisation?', *Social Science and Medicine,* 11 (1977)

Jenny, J. 'A Social Perspective on Need and Demand for Orthodontic Treatment', *International Dental Journal,* 25 (1975)

Jenny, J. *et al.* 'Parents' Satisfaction and Dissatisfaction with Their Children's Dentist', *Journal of Public Health Dentistry,* 33 (1973)

—— 'Explaining Variability in Caries Experience Using an Ecological Model', *Journal of Dental Research,* 53 (1974)

—— 'Dental Health Status of Third Grade Children and Their Families within the Context of a Community's Dental Health Care System', *Medical Care,* 13 (1975)

Jewson, N.D. 'Medical Knowledge and the Patronage System in Eighteenth Century England', *Sociology,* 8 (1974)

—— 'The Disappearance of the Sick-Man from Medical Cosmology, 1770-1870', *Sociology,* 10 (1976)

Johnson, J.E. 'Causes of Accidental Injuries to the Teeth and Jaws', *Journal of Public Health Dentistry,* 35 (1975)

Johnson, T. 'Imperialism and the Professions: Notes on the Development of Professional Occupations in Britain's Colonies and the New States' in P. Halmos (ed.), *Professionalisation and Social Change* (Sociological Review Monograph, University of Keele, 1973)

Judge, K. *Rationing Social Services: A Study of Resource Allocation and the Personal Social Services* (Heinemann, London, 1978)

Kasl, S.V. 'The Health Belief Model and Behavior Related to Chronic Illness', *Health Education Monograph,* 2 (1974)

Kasl, S.V. and Cobb, S. 'Health Behavior, Illness Behavior and Sick Role Behavior I', *Archives of Environmental Health,* 12 (1966)

Katz, R.V. 'Relationships Between Eight Orthodontic Indices and an

Oral Self-Image Satisfaction Scale', *American Journal of Orthodontics,* 73 (1978)

Kegeles, S.S. 'Some Motives for Seeking Preventive Dental Care', *Journal of the American Dental Association,* 67 (1963)

—— 'Adequate Oral Health: Blocks and Means by Which They May be Overcome' in W.E. Brown (ed.), *Oral Health, Dentistry, and the American Public* (University of Oklahoma Press, Norman, Oklahoma, 1974a)

—— 'Current Status of Preventive Dental Health Behavior in the Population', *Health Education Monograph,* 2 (1974b)

—— 'Public Acceptance of Dental Preventive Measures', *Journal of Preventive Dentistry,* 2 (1975)

Kelman, S. 'The Social Nature of the Definition: Problem in Health', *International Journal of Health Services,* 5 (1975)

Kesel, R.G. 'Dental Practice' in B.S. Hollinshead (ed.), *The Survey of Dentistry: The Final Report* (American Council on Education, Washington, 1961)

King, J.M. 'Patterns of Sugar Consumption in Early Infancy', *Community Dentistry and Oral Epidemiology,* 6 (1978)

Kirscht, J.P. 'Research Related to the Modification of Health Beliefs', *Health Education Monograph,* 2 (1974)

Kirscht, J.P. *et al.* 'Psychological and Social Factors as Predictors of Medical Behavior', *Medical Care,* 14 (1976)

Klegon, D. 'The Sociology of Professions: An Emerging Perspective', *Sociology of Work and Occupations,* 5 (1978)

Knafl, K. and Burkett, G. 'Professional Socialization in a Surgical Specialty: Acquiring Medical Judgment', *Social Science and Medicine,* 9 (1975)

Knowles, J.H. 'The Responsibility of the Individual' in J. Knowles (ed.), *Doing Better and Feeling Worse: Health in the United States* (W.W. Norton, New York, 1977)

Knutson, J.W. 'Controlling the Cost of Dental Health Care Insurance', *American Journal of Public Health,* 69 (1979)

Koch, G. and Martinsson, T. 'Socio-Odontologic Investigation of Schoolchildren with High and Low Caries Frequency. I. Socio-Economic Background', *Odontologisk Revy,* 21 (1970)

—— 'Socio-Odontologic Investigation of Schoolchildren with High and Low Caries Frequency. II. Parents' Opinion of Dietary Habits in Their Children', *Odontologisk Revy,* 22 (1971)

Kohn, R. and White, K.L. (eds.) *Health Care: An International Study* (Oxford University Press, London, 1976)

Koos, E.L. *The Health of Regionville* (Columbia University Press, New York, 1954)

Kostlan, J. 'Systems of Prevention in Dental Care', in WHO Regional Office for Europe, *Health Planning and Organization of Medical Care* (WHO, Copenhagen, 1972)

—— 'Dental Health Services in Europe: The Regional Role of the WHO' in G.L. Slack and B.A. Burt (eds.), *Dental Public Health: An Introduction to Community Dentistry* (John Wright and Sons, Bristol, 1974)

Krasner, D. 'Stress as a Distal Etiological Factor in Dental Disease', *Journal of Preventive Dentistry*, 5 (1978)

Kriesberg, L. 'The Relationship Between Socio-Economic Rank and Behavior', *Social Problems*, 10 (1963)

Kriesberg, L. and Treiman, B.R. 'Socioeconomic Status and the Utilization of Dentists' Services', *Journal of the American College of Dentists*, 27 (1960)

—— 'Preventive Utilization of Dentists' Services Among Teenagers', *Journal of the American College of Dentists*, 29 (1962)

Krilshevsky, D. 'Diet and Atherosclerosis', *American Journal of Pathology*, 84 (1976)

Kronenfeld, J.J. 'Self-Care as a Panacea for the Ills of the Health Care System: An Assessment', *Social Science and Medicine*, 13A (1979)

Kronus, C.L. 'Review of Jackson (ed.), Professions and Professionalization', *Sociology of Work and Occupations*, 1 (1974)

—— 'The Evolution of Occupational Power, an Historical Study of Task Boundaries Between Physicians and Pharmacists', *Sociology of Work and Occupations*, 3 (1976)

Kuhn T.S. *The Structure of Scientific Revolutions* (University of Chicago Press, Chicago, 1962)

Kumar, K. 'Industrialism and Post-Industrialism: Reflections on a Putative Transition', *Sociological Review*, 24 (1976)

Lalonde, M. *A New Perspective on the Health of Canadians – A Working Document* (Information Canada, Ottawa, 1974)

Lang, N.P. *et al.* 'Toothbrushing Frequency as it Relates to Plaque Development and Gingival Health', *Journal of Periodontology*, 44 (1973)

Langlie, J.K. 'Social Networks, Health Beliefs, and Preventive Health Behavior', *Journal of Health and Social Behavior*, 18 (1977)

Larkin, G.V. 'Medical Dominance and Control: Radiographers in the Division of Labour', *Sociological Review*, 26 (1978)

Leavitt, F. 'The Health Belief Model and Utilization of Ambulatory Care

Services', *Social Science and Medicine,* 13A (1979)

Lennon, M.A. 'Dental Care Delivery in the United Kingdom (England and Wales)' in J.I. Ingle and P. Blair (eds.), *International Dental Care Delivery Systems: Issues in Dental Health Policies* (Ballinger, Cambridge Mass., 1978)

Lennon, M.A. *et al.* 'Tooth Loss in a Nineteenth Century British Population', *Archives of Oral Biology,* 19 (1974)

Leske, G.S. *et al.* 'Comparison of Caries Prevalence of Children with Different Daily Toothbrushing Frequencies', *Community Dentistry and Oral Epidemiology,* 4 (1976)

Leverett, D.H. 'A Critical Examination of the Barriers to the Receipt of Dental Care', *Journal of Public Health Dentistry,* 35 (1975)

Leverett, D.H. and Jong, A. 'Variations in Use of Dental Care Facilities by Low-Income White and Black Populations', *Journal of the American Dental Association,* 80 (1970)

Lewis, M.H. 'Dental Care Delivery in Saskatchewan, Canada' in J.I. Ingle and P. Blair (eds.) *International Dental Care Delivery Systems: Issues in Dental Health Policies* (Ballinger, Cambridge Mass., 1978)

Lindhe, J. and Koch, G. 'The Effect of Supervised Oral Hygiene on the Gingivae of Children', *Journal of Periodontal Research,* 2 (1967)

Lindhe, J. *et al.* 'Effect of Proper Oral Hygiene on Gingivitis and Dental Caries in Swedish Schoolchildren', *Community Dentistry and Oral Epidemiology,* 3 (1975)

Linn, E.L. 'Oral Hygiene and Periodontal Disease: Implications for Dental Health Programs', *Journal of the American Dental Association,* 71 (1965)

—— 'Role Behaviors in Two Dental Clinics: A Trial of Nadel's Criteria', *Human Organization,* 26 (1967)

—— 'What Dental Patients Don't Know About Preventive Care', *Journal of Public Health Dentistry,* 34 (1974)

Löe, H. 'Progress in Improving Dental Health — A Discussion', *Journal of Public Health Dentistry,* 38 (1978)

Lomas, P. 'Ritualistic Elements in the Management of Childbirth', *British Journal of Medical Psychology,* 39 (1966)

Lotzkar, S. *et al.* 'Experimental Program in Expanded Functions for Dental Assistants; Phase 3: Experiment with Dental Teams', *Journal of the American Dental Association,* 82 (1971)

Lufkin, A.W. *A History of Dentistry* (Kimpton, London, 1948)

Lundquist, C. 'Tooth Mortality in Sweden: A Statistical Survey of Tooth Loss in the Swedish Population', *Acta Odontologica Scandinavica,* 25 (1967)

McCallum, C.A. 'Specialization in Dentistry', *International Dental Journal*, 28 (1978)

McCluggage, R.W. *A History of the American Dental Association* (Lakeside Press, Chicago, 1959)

McKeithen, E.J. 'The Patient's Image of the Dentist', *Journal of the American College of Dentists*, 33 (1966)

McKendrick, A.J.W. 'The Economics of Caries Prevention by Dental Hygienists', *Public Health*, 85 (1971)

McKeown, T. *The Role of Medicine: Dream, Mirage or Nemesis?* (Nuffield Provincial Hospitals Trust, London, 1976)

McKinlay, J.B. 'Some Approaches and Problems in the Study of the Use of Services – An Overview', *Journal of Health and Social Behavior*, 13 (1972)

—— 'On the Professional Regulation of Change' in P. Halmos (ed.), *Professionalisation and Social Change* (Sociological Review Monograph, University of Keele, 1973)

—— 'A Case for Refocussing Upstream – The Political Economy of Illness', *Proceedings of American Heart Association Conference*, Washington, 1974

—— 'The Business of Good Doctoring or Doctoring as Good Business: Reflections on Freidson's View of the Medical Game', *International Journal of Health Services*, 7 (1977)

—— 'The Political Economy of Dental Illness and Dental Care' (Unpublished Paper Presented to IADR Symposium, Wellington, New Zealand, 1978)

McKinlay, J.B. and McKinlay, S.M. 'The Questionable Contribution of Medical Measures to the Decline of Mortality in the United States in the Twentiety Century', *Milbank Memorial Fund Quarterly (Health and Society)*, 55 (1977)

Mahler, H. 'Health – A Demystification of Medical Technology', *Lancet*, 2 (1978)

Mandel, I.D. 'Effectiveness of Biomedical and Biosocial Research on Improving Oral Health', *Journal of Public Health Dentistry*, 38 (1978)

Manning, J.E. 'Dental Ancillaries for the Seventies', *British Dental Journal*, 131 (1970)

Mansbridge, J.N. 'The Influence of Social and Economic Conditions on the Prevalance of Dental Caries', *Archives of Oral Biology*, 1 (1959)

—— 'The Effects of Oral Hygiene and Sweet Consumption on the Prevalence of Dental Caries', *British Dental Journal*, 109 (1960)

Mapes, R.E.A. 'Physicians' Drug Innovation and Relinquishment', *Social Science and Medicine*, 11 (1977)

Marbach, J.J. and Lipton, J.A. 'Aspects of Illness Behavior in Patients with Facial Pain', *Journal of the American Dental Association,* 96 (1978)

Markkula, J. *et al.* 'Conceptions of Finnish People About the Etiology and Prevention of Dental Caries and Periodontal Disorders', *Community Dentistry and Oral Epidemiology,* 5 (1977)

Martens, L.V. *et al.* 'New Dental Care Concepts: Perceptions of Dentists and Dental Students', *American Journal of Public Health,* 61 (1971)

Marthaler, T.M. 'Epidemiological and Clinical Dental Findings in Relation to Intake of Carbohydrates', *Caries Research,* 1 (1967)

—— 'Decrease of DMF-Levels 4 Years After the Introduction of a Caries Preventive Program. Observations in 5819 Schoolchildren of 20 Communities', *Helvitica Odontologica Acta,* 16 (1972a)

—— 'Reduction in Caries, Gingivitis and Calculus After Eight Years of Preventive Measures – Observations in 7 Communities', *Helvitica Odontologica Acta,* 16 (1972b)

Marthaler, T.M. *et al.* 'Caries-Preventive Salt Fluoridation', *Caries Research,* 12 (Suppl. 1) (1978)

Martinsson, T. 'Socio-Odontologic Investigation of School Children with High and Low Caries Frequency', *Odontologisk Revy,* 24 (Suppl. 24) (1973)

Maxwell, R. *Health Care, the Growing Dilemma: Needs versus Resources in Western Europe, the U.S. and the U.S.S.R.* (McKinsey, New York, 1974)

Mechanic, D. 'Sex, Illness, Illness Behavior, and the Use of Health Services', *Social Science and Medicine,* 12B (1978)

Menzies Campbell, J. *From a Trade to a Profession: Byways in Dental History* (Private Publication, Alva, 1958)

—— 'An Outline of Dental History', *British Dental Journal,* 129 (1970)

Meskin, L.H. *et al.* 'Effectiveness of Community Preventive Programs on Improving Oral Health', *Journal of Public Health Dentistry,* 38 (1978)

Metz, A.S. and Richards, L.G. 'Children's Preventive Visits to the Dentist: The Relative Importance of Socio-Economic Factors and Parents' Preventive Visits', *Journal of the American College of Dentists,* 34 (1967)

Meyers, H.B. 'The Medical-Industrial Complex', *Fortune,* 81 (1970)

Michel, C. 'The General Causes of the Increase in Sickness Insurance Expenditure on Medical Care', *International Social Security Review,* 27 (1974)

Miller, A. 'The Wages of Neglect: Death and Disease in the American Workplace', *American Journal of Public Health,* 65 (1975)

Miller, L. 'Healthy, Wealthy, and Wise: An Essay Review of "Doing Better and Feeling Worse: Health in the United States" J. Knowles (ed.)', *Social Science and Medicine,* 12 (1978)

Millerson, G.L. *The Qualifying Associations* (Routledge and Kegan Paul, London, 1964)

Moen, B.D. and Poetsch, W.E. 'More Preventive Care, Less Tooth Repair', *Journal of the American Dental Association,* 81 (1970)

Montoya, R. *et al.* 'Minority Dental School Graduates: Do They Serve Minority Communities?', *American Journal of Public Health,* 68 (1978)

Moosbruker, J.M. and Jong, A. 'Racial Similarities and Differences in Family Dental Care Patterns', *Public Health Reports,* 84 (1969)

Morris, A.L. 'Dentistry: Retrospect and Prospect', *Journal of the American Dental Association,* 87 (1973)

Murtomaa, H. and Ainamo, J. 'Conceptions of Finnish People About Their Periodontal Situation', *Community Dentistry and Oral Epidemiology,* 5 (1977)

Myrberg, N. and Thilander, B. 'Orthodontic Need of Treatment of Swedish Schoolchildren from Objective and Subjective Aspects', *Scandinavian Journal of Dental Research,* 81 (1973)

Nathanson, C.A. 'Sex Roles as Variables in Preventive Health Behaviour', *Journal of Community Health,* 3 (1977)

—— 'Sex Roles as Variables in the Interpretation of Morbidity Data: A Methodological Critique', *International Journal of Epidemiology,* 7 (1978)

Navarro, V. 'The Political Economy of Medical Care: An Explanation of the Composition, Nature and Functions of the Present Health Sector in the United States', *International Journal of Health Services,* 5 (1975)

Newbrun, E. and Frostell, G. 'Sugar Restriction and Substitution for Caries Prevention', *Caries Research,* 12 (1978)

Nikias, M.K. *et al.* 'Comparisons of Poverty and Nonpoverty Groups on Dental Status, Needs and Practices', *Journal of Public Health Dentistry,* 35 (1975)

—— 'Oral Health Status in Relation to Socioeconomic and Ethnic Characteristics of Urban Adults in the USA', *Community Dentistry and Oral Epidemiology,* 5 (1977)

Nippert, R.P. 'Dentists' Work and Dental Health Needs' (Unpublished Paper Presented at IX World Congress of Sociology, Uppsala, 1978)

Numbers, R.L. *Almost Persuaded: American Physicians and Compulsory Health Insurance, 1912-1920* (Johns Hopkins University Press,

Baltimore, 1978)

O'Mullane, D.M. and Robinson, M.E. 'The Distribution of Dentists and the Uptake of Dental Treatment by Schoolchildren in England', *Community Dentistry and Oral Epidemiology,* 5 (1977)

O'Shea, R.M. 'Characteristics of Dental Practice' in N.D. Richards and L.K. Cohen (eds.), *Social Sciences and Dentistry: A Critical Bibliography* (Sijthoff, The Hague, 1971a)

— 'Dentistry as an Organization and Institution', *Milbank Memorial Fund Quarterly,* 49 (1971b)

O'Shea, R.M. and Gray, S.B. 'Dental Patients' Attitudes and Behavior Concerning Prevention', *Public Health Reports,* 83 (1968)

O'Shea, R.M. *et al.* 'Sociologic Perspective on the Dental Student', *Journal of Dental Education,* 30 (1966)

Ozonoff, V.V. and Ozonoff, D. 'Steps Toward a Radical Analysis of Health Care: Problems and Prospects', *International Journal of Health Services,* 5 (1975)

Parry, N. and Parry, J. 'Professionalism and Unionism: Aspects of Class Conflict in the N.H.S.', *Sociological Review,* 25 (1977)

Parsons, T. 'The Sick Role and the Role of the Physician Reconsidered', *Milbank Memorial Fund Quarterly (Health and Society),* 53 (1975)

Payne, A.M.-M. 'Innovation Out of Unity', *Milbank Memorial Fund Quarterly,* 43 (1965)

Pelton, W.J. *et al.* 'Tooth Morbidity in Adults', *Journal of the American Dental Association,* 49 (1954)

Petterson, E.O. and Littleton, P.A. 'Preventive and Community Dentistry in the Dental Schools of the U.S.', *Journal of Public Health Dentistry,* 31 (1971)

Pflanz, M. 'German Health Insurance: The Evolution and Current Problems of the Pioneer System', *International Journal of Health Services,* 1 (1971)

Pineault, R. 'The Effect of Prepaid Group Practice on Physicians' Utilization Behavior', *Medical Care,* 14 (1976)

Plasschaert, A.J.M. *et al.* 'An Epidemiologic Survey of Periodontal Disease in Dutch Adults', *Community Dentistry and Oral Epidemiology,* 6 (1978)

Posner, T. 'Magical Elements in Orthodox Medicine: Diabetes as a Medical Thought System' in R. Dingwall *et al.* (eds.), *Health Care and Health Knowledge* (Croom Helm, London, 1977)

Pratt, L. 'How Do Patients Learn About Disease?', *Social Problems,* 4 (1956)

— 'The Relationship of Socioeconomic Status to Health', *American*

Journal of Public Health, 61 (1971)

Quarantelli, E.L. 'The Dental Student Image of the Dentist-Patient Relationship', *American Journal of Public Health,* 51 (1961)

Rajala, A. *et al.* 'Utilization of Dental Care in a Finnish Industrial Population', *Community Dentistry and Oral Epidemiology,* 6 (1978)

Ramirez, A. *et al.* 'Use of Simulated Experience in Teaching Community Dentistry', *Journal of Dental Education,* 31 (1967)

Rayner, J.F. and Cohen, L.K. 'Behavioral Factors in Oral Hygiene' in H.J.V. Goldberg and L.W. Ripa (eds.), *Oral Hygiene and Oral Health* (Charles C. Thomas, Springfield Ill., 1977)

Reiss, M.L. *et al.* 'Behavioral Community Psychology: Encouraging Low-Income Patients to Seek Dental Care for Their Children', *Journal of Applied Behavioral Analysis,* 9 (1976)

Renaud, M. 'On the Structural Constraints to State Intervention in Health', *International Journal of Health Services,* 5 (1975)

Retief, D.H. *et al.* 'Dental Caries and Sugar Intake in South African Pupils of 16 to 17 Years in 4 Ethnic Groups', *British Dental Journal,* 138 (1975)

Revere, P. *Dentistry and Its Victims* (St. Martin's Press, New York, 1970)

Rhee, S. 'Factors Determining the Quality of Physician Performance in Patient Care', *Medical Care,* 14 (1976)

—— 'Relative Importance of Physicians' Personal and Situational Characteristics for the Quality of Patient Care', *Journal of Health and Social Behaviour,* 18 (1977)

Richards, N.D. 'Dentistry in England in the 1840's: The First Indications of a Movement Towards Professionalization',*Medical History,* 12 (1968)

—— 'Dentistry in Great Britain: Some Sociologic Perspectives', *Milbank Memorial Fund Quarterly,* 49 (1971a)

—— 'From Trader to Professional: The Evolution of the Dentist and Dental Services 1840-1921', *Social History of Medicine Bulletin,* 4 (1971b)

—— 'Methods and Effectiveness of Health Education: The Past, Present and Future of Social Scientific Development', *Social Science and Medicine,* 9 (1975)

Richards, N.D. *et al.* 'A Survey of the Dental Health and Attitudes Towards Dentistry in Two Communities: Part I. Sociological Data', *British Dental Journal,* 118 (1965)

Richardson, B.D. *et al.* 'Total Sucrose Intake and Dental Caries in Black and White South African Children of 1-6 Years. Part I. Sucrose Intake', *Journal of the Dental Association of South Africa,* 33 (1978a)

— 'Total Sucrose Intake and Dental Caries in Black and White South African Children of 1-6 years. Part II. Dental Caries and Sucrose Intake', *Journal of the Dental Association of South Africa,* 33 (1978b)

Ringelberg, M.L. and Tonascia, J.A. 'A Regression Model Analysis of Longitudinal Dental Caries Data', *Community Dentistry and Oral Epidemiology,* 4 (1976)

Ringen, K. 'The "New Ferment" in National Health Policies: The Case of Norway's Nutrition and Food Policy', *Social Science and Medicine,* 13C (1979)

Rise, J. and Helöe, L.A. 'Oral Conditions and Need for Dental Treatment in an Elderly Population in Northern Norway', *Community Dentistry and Oral Epidemiology,* 6 (1978)

Robertson, L.S. 'Behavioral Research and Strategies in Public Health: A Demur', *Social Science and Medicine,* 9 (1975)

Roder, D.M. 'The Dental Health and Habits of South Australian Children From Different Socio-Economic Environments', *Australian Dental Journal,* 16 (1971)

— 'The Effect of Treatment Provided by Dentists and Therapists in the South Australian School Dental Service', *Australian Dental Journal,* 18 (1973)

Rodman, H. 'Culture of Poverty: The Rise and Fall of a Concept', *Sociological Review,* 25 (1977)

Roemer, M.I. 'Social Security for Medical Care: Is it Justified in Developing Countries?', *International Journal of Health Services,* 1 (1971)

Rosen, H.M. *et al.* 'Capitation in Dentistry: A Quasi-Experimental Evaluation', *Medical Care,* 15 (1977)

Rosenbaum, S. 'Social Services Manpower', *Social Trends,* 2 (1971)

Rosenstock, I.M. 'Why People Use Health Services', *Milbank Memorial Fund Quarterly,* 44 (1966)

Rosenthal, G. and Fox, D.M. 'A Right to What?: Toward Adequate Minimum Standards for Personal Health Services', *Milbank Memorial Fund Quarterly (Health and Society),* 56 (1978)

Roskies, E. 'Sex, Culture and Illness — An Overview', *Social Science and Medicine,* 12B (1978)

Roth, J.A. 'Professionalism: The Sociologist's Decoy', *Sociology of Work and Occupations,* 1 (1974)

Rothstein, R.J. *The History of Dental Laboratories and Their Contributions to Dentistry* (Lippincott, Philadelphia, 1958)

Rothstein, W.G. 'Professionalization and Employer Demands: The Cases

of Homeopathy and Psychoanalysis in the United States' in P.
Halmos (ed.), *Professionalisation and Social Change* (Sociological
Review Monograph, University of Keele, 1973)

Russell, A.L. 'International Nutrition Surveys: A Summary of
Preliminary Dental Findings', *Journal of Dental Research*, 42 (1963)

Russell, A.L. and Ayers, P. 'Periodontal Disease and Socioeconomic
Status in Birmingham, Alabama', *American Journal of Public Health*,
50 (1960)

Salber, E.J. *et al.* 'Utilization of Services for Preventable Disease: A Case
Study of Dental Care in a Southern Rural Area of the United States',
International Journal of Epidemiology, 7 (1978)

Samuelson, G. *et al.* 'An Epidemiological Study of Child Health and
Nutrition in a Northern Swedish County: VI. Relationship Between
General and Oral Health, Food Habits and Socio-Economic
Condition', *American Journal of Clinical Nutrition*, 24 (1971)

Scarrott, D.M. 'Attitudes to Dentists', *British Dental Journal*, 127 (1969)

Scheff, T.J. 'Decision Rules, Types of Errors, and Their Consequences
in Medical Diagnosis'. *Behavioral Science*, 8 (1963)

—— 'Typification in the Diagnostic Practice of Rehabilitation Agencies'
in M.B. Sussman (ed.), *Sociology and Rehabilitation* (American
Sociological Association, Washington, 1966)

Scheinin, A. *et al.* 'Turku Sugar Studies I', *Acta Odontologica
Scandinavica*, 32 (1974)

Schoen, M.H. 'Dental Care and the Health Maintenance Organization
Concept', *Milbank Memorial Fund Quarterly* (Health and Society),
53 (1975)

—— 'Dental Care Delivery in the U.S.' in J.I. Ingle and P. Blair (eds.),
*International Dental Care Delivery Systems: Issues in Dental
Health Policies* (Ballinger, Cambridge Mass., 1978)

Schonfeld, H.K. 'Periodontal Diseases in Association with Unmet Dental
Needs', *American Journal of Public Health*, 53 (1963)

—— 'Origin and Growth of Dental Group Practice and Closed Panels',
New York State Dental Journal, 36 (1970)

Segall, A. 'Sociocultural Variation in Sick Role Behavioral
Expectations', *Social Science and Medicine*, 10 (1976)

Seifert, I. *et al.* 'Evaluation of Psychologic Factors in Geriatric Denture
Patients', *Journal of Prosthetic Dentistry*, 12 (1962)

Shannon, I.L. 'Concentration of Sugars in Commercial Baby Foods',
Journal of Dentistry for Children, 45 (1978)

Shapiro, A.K. 'A Contribution to the History of the Placebo Effect',
Behavioral Science, 5 (1960)

Sheiham, A. 'The Prevalence and Severity of Periodontal Disease in British Populations', *British Dental Journal,* 126 (1969)
—— 'An Evaluation of the Success of Dental Care in the United Kingdom', *British Dental Journal,* 135 (1973)
—— 'Is There a Scientific Basis for Six-Monthly Dental Examinations?', *Lancet,* 2 (1977)
Sheiham, A. and Hobdell, M.H. 'Decayed, Missing, and Filled Teeth in British Adult Populations', *British Dental Journal,* 126 (1969)
Sheiham, A. and Striffler, D.F. 'A Comparison of Four Epidemiological Methods for Assessing Periodontal Disease I. Population Findings', *Journal of Periodontal Research,* 5 (1970)
Shryock, R.H. *The Development of Modern Medicine: An Interpretation of the Social and Scientific Factors Involved* (Gollancz, London, 1948)
Shuval, J.T. 'Sex Role Differentiation in the Professions: The Case of Israeli Dentists', *Journal of Health and Social Behavior,* 11 (1970)
—— 'Levels of Professionalism in a Dual System of Dental Care', *Journal of Public Health Dentistry,* 31 (1971)
Silversin, J.B. *et al.* 'The Teaching and Practice of Some Clinical Aspects of Endodontics in Great Britain', *Journal of Dentistry,* 3 (1975)
—— 'A Multiple Regression Approach to Predicting Preventive Behavior in Dental Practice', *Journal of Dental Education,* 41 (1977)
Skogedal, O. and Helöe, L.A. 'Public Opinions on Dentists in Norway', *Community Dentistry and Oral Epidemiology,* 7 (1979)
Smith, J.P. 'The Pain Dysfunction Syndrome. Why Females?', *Journal of Dentistry,* 4 (1976)
Smith, L.W. *et al.* 'Teachers as Models in Programs for School Dental Health; An Evaluation of the "Toothkeeper" ', *Journal of Public Health Dentistry,* 35 (1975)
Sognnaes, R.F. 'A Survey of Dental Caries in Greece', *New York State Dental Journal,* 15 (1949)
Stadt, Z.M. 'Socio-Economic Status and Dental Experience of 3911 Five Year Old Natives of Contra Costa County, California', *Journal of Public Health Dentistry,* 27 (1967)
Stamm, J.W. 'An Overview of Dental Care Delivery Systems in Canada', *International Dental Journal,* 28 (1978)
Stamm, J.W. *et al.* 'An Evaluation of the "Toothkeeper" Program in Vermont', *Journal of Public Health Dentistry,* 35 (1975)
Stevenson, G. 'Social Relations of Production and Consumption in the Human Service Occupations', *International Journal of Health Services,* 8 (1978)

Stoeckle, J.D. *et al.* 'On Going to See the Doctor, the Contributions of the Patient to the Decision to Seek Medical Aid', *Journal of Chronic Diseases,* 16 (1963)

Strauss, A. *Psychiatric Ideologies and Institutions* (Free Press, Glencoe, 1964)

Suchman, E.A. 'Health Attitudes and Behavior', *Archives of Environmental Health,* 20 (1970)

Suchman, E.A. and Rothman, A.A. 'The Utilization of Dental Services', *Milbank Memorial Fund Quarterly,* 49 (1969)

Sudnow, D. 'Normal Crimes: Sociological Features of the Penal Code in a Public Defender's Office', *Social Problems,* 12 (1965)

Suher, T. and Savara, B.S. 'Incidence of Dental Caries in Children 1 to 6 Years of Age', *Journal of Dental Research,* 33 (1954)

Sutton, R. and Sheiham, A. 'The Factual Basis for Health Education. A Review', *Health Education Journal,* 33 (1974)

Tash, R.H. *et al.* 'Testing a Preventive-Symptomatic Theory of Dental Health Behavior', *American Journal of Public Health,* 59 (1969)

Taylor, D.G. *et al.* 'A Social Indicator of Access to Medical Care', *Journal of Health and Social Behavior,* 16 (1975)

Taylor, P.J. 'Some International Trends in Sickness Absence, 1950-1968', *British Medical Journal,* 4 (1969)

Terris, M. 'Epidemiology of Cirrhosis of the Liver: National Mortality Data', *American Journal of Public Health,* 57 (1967)

— 'The Epidemiologic Revolution, National Health Insurance and the Role of Health Departments', *American Journal of Public Health,* 66 (1976)

Thomson, P.L. 'Sweetened Drinks as a Source of Sugar Intake in Selected Teenagers in South-East England', *Community Dentistry and Oral Epidemiology,* 5 (1977)

Toverud, G. 'The Influence of War and Post-War Conditions on the Teeth of Norwegian School Children. III. Discussion of Food Supply and Dental Condition in Norway and Other European Countries', *Milbank Memorial Fund Quarterly,* 35 (1957)

Tudor Hart, J. 'The Inverse Care Law', *Lancet,* 1 (1971)

— 'Primary Care in the Industrial Areas of Britain: Evolution and Current Problems', *International Journal of Health Services,* 2 (1972)

Twaddle, A.C. 'Illness and Deviance', *Social Science and Medicine,* 7 (1973)

USPHS, 'Periodontal Disease in Adults, U.S. 1960-1962', *National Center for Health Statistics (Series 11),* 12 (1965a)

— 'Selected Dental Findings in Adults by Age, Race, and Sex – U.S.,

1960-1962' *National Center for Health Statistics (Series 11),* 7 (1965b)
— 'Decayed, Missing, and Filled Teeth in Adults, U.S., 1960-1962',
National Center for Health Statistics (Series 11), 23 (1967a)
— 'Total Tooth Loss of Teeth in Adults, U.S., 1960-1962', *National
Center for Health Statistics (Series 11),* 27 (1967b)
— 'Need for Dental Care Among Adults, U.S., 1960-1962', *National
Center for Health Statistics (Series 11),* 36 (1970)
— 'Decayed, Missing, and Filled Teeth Among Children', *National
Center for Health Statistics (Series 11),* 106 (1971)
— 'Periodontal Disease and Oral Hygiene Among Children', *National
Center for Health Statistics (Series 11),* 117 (1972)
— 'An Assessment of the Occlusion of the Teeth of Children 6-11
Years', *National Center for Health Statistics (Series 11),* 130 (1973)
— 'Decayed, Missing, and Filled Teeth Among Youths 12-17 Years',
National Center for Health Statistics (Series 11), 144 (1974a)
— 'Periodontal Disease Among Youths 12-17 Years', *National Center
for Health Statistics (Series 11),* 141 (1974b)
— 'An Assessment of the Occlusion of the Teeth of Youths, 12-17
Years', *National Center for Health Statistics (Series 11),* 162 (1977)
— 'Basic Data on Dental Examination Findings of Persons 1-74 Years',
National Center for Health Statistics (Series 11), 214 (1979)
Vayda, E. 'When is Surgery Indicated? A Book Review', *Milbank
Memorial Fund Quarterly (Health and Society),* 55 (1977)
Vogan, W.I. 'Dental Knowledge and Attitudes', *British Dental Journal,*
128 (1970)
Vutov, M. 'Some Characteristic Features of the History of Stomatology
in Bulgaria', *International Dental Journal,* 19 (1969)
Waddington, I. 'The Role of the Hospital in the Development of Modern
Medicine: A Sociological Analysis', *Sociology,* 7 (1973)
— 'The Development of Medical Ethics — A Sociological Analysis',
Medical History, 19 (1975)
— 'General Practitioners and Consultants in Early Nineteenth Century
England: The Sociology of an Intra-Professional Conflict' in J.
Woodward and N.D. Richards (eds.), *Health Care and Popular
Medicine in Nineteenth Century England: Essays in the Social
History of Medicine* (Croom Helm, London 1977)
Waldman, H.B. 'Participation of Dentists in the Activities of their Local
Societies', *Journal of Public Health Dentistry,* 31 (1971)
Waldron, I. 'Increased Prescribing of Valium, Librium, and Other Drugs
— An Example of the Influence of Economic and Social Factors',
International Journal of Health Services, 7 (1977)

Walker, R.O. 'The Socialization of Dentistry', *British Dental Journal,* 122 (1967)

Wan, T.T.H. and Yates, A.S. 'Prediction of Dental Services Utilization: A Multivariate Approach', *Inquiry,* 12 (1975)

Wandelt, S. 'Statistical Survey of the Relation Between Sugar Consumption and Dental Caries', *Nutrition Abstracts Review,* 39 (1969)

Wardwell, W.I. 'Limited, Marginal, and Quasi-Practitioners' in H.E. Freeman *et al.* (eds.), *Handbook of Medical Sociology,* 2nd edn. (Prentice-Hall, Englewood Cliffs, N.J., 1972)

Wechsler, H. *et al.* 'Location and Practice Busyness: Maldistribution of Dental Services in New York State', *New York State Dental Journal,* 38 (1972)

Weinberg, L.A. 'An Evaluation of Stress in Temperomandibular Joint Dysfunction-Pain Syndrome', *Journal of Prosthetic Dentistry,* 38 (1977)

Whitehead, F.E. 'Trends in Certificated Sickness Absence', *Social Trends,* 2 (1971)

Wilding, G.V. and Wilding, P. 'Social Values, Social Class and Social Policy', *Social and Economic Adminstration,* 6 (1972)

Wilkinson, R.C. 'Dear David Ennals . . . An Open Letter', *New Society,* 38 (1976)

Willcocks, A.J. and Richards, N.D. 'Dental Manpower and Dentistry as an Institution' in N.D. Richards and L.K. Cohen (eds.), *Social Sciences and Dentistry: A Critical Bibliography* (Sijthoff, The Hague, 1971)

Williams, A.F. *et al.* 'Dental Manpower in an Urban Area', *Medical Care,* 7 (1969)

Williams, T.F. *et al.* 'The Clinical Picture of Diabetes Control, Studies in Four Settings', *American Journal of Public Health,* 57 (1967)

Wilson, R.W. and White, E.L. 'Changes in Morbidity, Disability, and Utilization Differentials Between the Poor and the Nonpoor: Data from the Health Interview Survey: 1964 and 1973', *Medical Care,* 15 (1977)

Winikoff, B. 'Nutrition and Food Policy: The Approaches of Norway and the U.S.', *American Journal of Public Health,* 67 (1977)

Wolinsky, F.D. 'Assessing the Effects of Predisposing, Enabling, and Illness-Morbidity Characteristics on Health Service Utilization', *Journal of Health and Social Behavior,* 19 (1978)

Wolock, I. and Wellin, E. 'Social Organisation of the Dental Profession in a Small City', *Milbank Memorial Fund Quarterly,* 49 (1971)

WHO, 'Organization of Dental Public Health Services', *Technical Report*

Series, 298 (1965)
—— 'Planning and Evaluation of Public Dental Health Services',
Technical Report Series, 589 (1976)
—— 'Epidemiology, Etiology, and Prevention of Periodontal Diseases',
Technical Report Series, 621 (1978)
WHO Regional Office for Europe, *Health Planning and Organization of Medical Care* (WHO, Copenhagen, 1972)
—— *Chronic Diseases* (WHO, Copenhagen, 1973)
Yassin, I. and Low, T. 'Caries Prevalence in Different Racial Groups of Schoolchildren in West Malaysia', *Community Dentistry and Oral Epidemiology,* 3 (1975)
Young, W.O. 'Dentistry Looks Toward the Twenty-First Century' in W.E. Brown (ed.), *Oral Health, Dentistry, and the American Public* (University of Oklahoma Press, Norman, Oklahoma, 1974)
Young, W.O. and Smith L. 'The Nature and Organization of Dental Practice' in H.E. Freeman *et al.* (eds.), *Handbook of Medical Sociology* 2nd edn. (Prentice-Hall, Englewood Cliffs, N.J., 1972)
Young, W.O. and Striffler, D.F. *The Dentist, His Practice and His Community* 2nd edn. (W.B. Saunders, Philadelphia, 1969)
Zadik, D. 'Epidemiology of Dental Caries in 5-Year-Old Children in Israel', *Community Dentistry and Oral Epidemiology,* 6 (1978)
Zola, I.K. 'Culture and Symptoms: An Analysis of Patients Presenting Symptoms', *American Sociological Review,* 31 (1966)

SUBJECT INDEX

access 52, 55, 65, 72, 77-8, 83-4, 92,
    95-6, 102, 131-2, 136, 145, 148
age 69, 78-9, 88, 101, 109-10, 113,
    127-8, 140; and demographic
    structure 21-2; and dental services
    28n12, 44, 65-8, 94, 112-14, 125,
    136, 149, 151n8, 151n12; and
    diet 44, 64-5; and health 24, 63-6,
    70, 75-6, 80n3, 116, 118n6; and
    'social' age 65, 79; and tooth loss
    23, 64-5, 68, 117
ageing 24, 26, 63-6
American Dental Association (ADA)
    28n1, 45n13
American Medical Association
    (AMA) 19, 31, 57, 60n10
American Stomatological Association
    105
apothecary 29, 32-5, 39, 43, 44n1,
    48
area of residence 46n15, 56, 70-1,
    84, 101
Australia 24, 49, 63
availability 50, 72, 117

barber 15, 29-30, 33, 48
barriers 95, 128; economic 72, 92,
    99n10; pain 92; social 73, 99n10,
    140
biological factors 63-9, 74, 79, 81,
    121
bleeding gums 101-2, *see also* gingi-
    vitis, periodontal disease
'blood-and-vulcanite' 108
British Dental Association (BDA) 55

Canada 46n16, 49, 52, 69, 151n11
Chadwick, Edwin 43, 63
China 45n6
client 39; as consumer 26, 54-5, 95,
    98n2, 133; *see also* patient
clientele 107, 130, 150
clinical model 120-5, 129, 133-5,
    149-50
clinical science 42, 44, 61, 138; and
    autonomy 38-40, 45n12, 143;
    and judgement 105-6, 115, 125,
    127, 134

clinics 44, 54, 71
colleague networks 50-1, 119n11;
    and Delta Sigma Delta 60n5
colleague relationships 38, 40, 51,
    143, 150
community dentistry 134
Company of Grocers 33
compliance 92-3
cultural factors 20, 57, 59, 65, 71,
    74, 76, 82, 99n10, 106, 109-10,
    123, 125, 131, 139, 145; atti-
    tudes: to dental care 72, 78, 97,
    to health 21, to patients 73;
    expectations 65-6, 83-4, 108,
    130, 132, 137n7; lay culture 43,
    67, 80, 90-7, 100-3, 116-18,
    144-5; life-style 22, 45n10,
    46n16, 70, 75, 81, 83-91, 96-8,
    103, 145-6, 150; professional
    culture 45n11, 90, 99n6, 100-10,
    117-18, 120, 150; public image of
    dentistry 13-15, 23, 28n9, 104,
    111, 115, 120-6, 129, 143; values
    31, 45, 64, 84, 98, 140; *see also*
    health beliefs
culture lag 101-2
culture of poverty 99n10

dental auxiliaries 17, 23, 25, 28n11,
    35, 37, 45n7, 49, 50, 55, 58,
    59n4, 109, 115, 131, 133, 148,
    151n11
dental care system 66, 71, 75, 78, 83,
    95, 112, 127, 132, 135-6, 143-6,
    149; treatment-oriented 24,
    127-8, 131, 136, 148; *see also*
    organisation and delivery of care
dental caries 22, 24, 65, 70, 76,
    80n2, 81, 84-5, 93, 97, 100-3,
    112, 126, 142, 146-7; incidence
    64, 87, 98n5; prevalence 75;
    research 28n10, 116; susceptibil-
    ity 68-9, 77
dental chairside assistants 23, 59n3
dental dressers 35, 49, 59n2
dental education 14, 25-6, 28n12,
    33, 35, 103, 106-7, 123, 129,
    133-4, 146, 148

AUTHOR INDEX